50% OFF
Online EMT Prep Course!

By Mometrix

Dear Customer,

We consider it an honor and a privilege that you chose our EMT Study Guide. As a way of showing our appreciation and to help us better serve you, we are offering **50% off our online EMT Prep Course**. Many EMT courses are needlessly expensive and don't deliver enough value. With our course, you get access to the best EMT prep material, and **you only pay half price**.

We have structured our online course to perfectly complement your printed study guide. The EMT Prep Course contains **in-depth lessons** that cover all the most important topics, **20+ video reviews** that explain difficult concepts, over **450 practice questions** to ensure you feel prepared, and more than **550 digital flashcards**, so you can study while you're on the go.

Online EMT Prep Course

Topics Included:	Course Features:
• Preparatory	• EMT Study Guide
o EMS Systems	o Get content that complements our best-selling study guide.
o Research	
• Medical Terminology	• Full-Length Practice Tests
o Life Span Development	o With over 450 practice questions, you can test yourself again and again.
o Public Health	
• Pharmacology	• Mobile Friendly
o Principles of Pharmacology	o If you need to study on the go, the course is easily accessible from your mobile device.
o Medication Administration	
• Assessment	• EMT Flashcards
o Primary Assessment	o Our course includes a flashcard mode with over 350 content cards to help you study.
o History Taking	

To receive this discount, visit us at mometrix.com/university/emt or simply scan this QR code with your smartphone. At the checkout page, enter the discount code: **EMT50off**

If you have any questions or concerns, please contact us at support@mometrix.com.

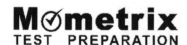

FREE Study Skills Videos/DVD Offer

Dear Customer,

Thank you for your purchase from Mometrix! We consider it an honor and a privilege that you have purchased our product and we want to ensure your satisfaction.

As part of our ongoing effort to meet the needs of test takers, we have developed a set of Study Skills Videos that we would like to give you for <u>FREE</u>. These videos cover our *best practices* for getting ready for your exam, from how to use our study materials to how to best prepare for the day of the test.

All that we ask is that you email us with feedback that would describe your experience so far with our product. Good, bad, or indifferent, we want to know what you think!

To get your FREE Study Skills Videos, you can use the **QR code** below, or send us an **email** at <u>studyvideos@mometrix.com</u> with *FREE VIDEOS* in the subject line and the following information in the body of the email:

- The name of the product you purchased.
- Your product rating on a scale of 1-5, with 5 being the highest rating.
- Your feedback. It can be long, short, or anything in between. We just want to know your impressions and experience so far with our product. (Good feedback might include how our study material met your needs and ways we might be able to make it even better. You could highlight features that you found helpful or features that you think we should add.)

If you have any questions or concerns, please don't hesitate to contact me directly.

Thanks again!

Sincerely,

Jay Willis
Vice President
<u>jay.willis@mometrix.com</u>
1-800-673-8175

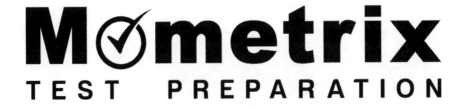

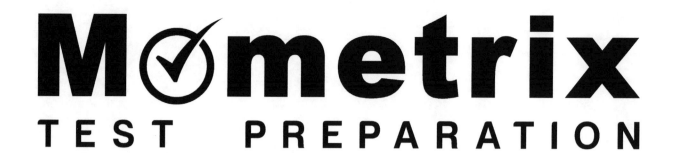

EMT

Book
2022-2023

NREMT Study Guide Secrets Test Prep

Full-Length Practice Exam

Detailed Answer
Explanations

4th Edition

Written and edited by Mometrix Test Prep

Printed in the United States of America

This paper meets the requirements of ANSI/NISO Z39.48-1992 (Permanence of Paper).

Mometrix offers volume discount pricing to institutions. For more information or a price quote, please contact our sales department at sales@mometrix.com or 888-248-1219.

Mometrix Media LLC is not affiliated with or endorsed by any official testing organization. All organizational and test names are trademarks of their respective owners.

Paperback
ISBN 13: 978-1-5167-2019-4
ISBN 10: 1-5167-2019-9

DEAR FUTURE EXAM SUCCESS STORY

First of all, **THANK YOU** for purchasing Mometrix study materials!

Second, congratulations! You are one of the few determined test-takers who are committed to doing whatever it takes to excel on your exam. **You have come to the right place.** We developed these study materials with one goal in mind: to deliver you the information you need in a format that's concise and easy to use.

In addition to optimizing your guide for the content of the test, we've outlined our recommended steps for breaking down the preparation process into small, attainable goals so you can make sure you stay on track.

We've also analyzed the entire test-taking process, identifying the most common pitfalls and showing how you can overcome them and be ready for any curveball the test throws you.

Standardized testing is one of the biggest obstacles on your road to success, which only increases the importance of doing well in the high-pressure, high-stakes environment of test day. Your results on this test could have a significant impact on your future, and this guide provides the information and practical advice to help you achieve your full potential on test day.

Your success is our success

We would love to hear from you! If you would like to share the story of your exam success or if you have any questions or comments in regard to our products, please contact us at **800-673-8175** or **support@mometrix.com**.

Thanks again for your business and we wish you continued success!

Sincerely,
The Mometrix Test Preparation Team

Need more help? Check out our flashcards at:
http://MometrixFlashcards.com/EMT

TABLE OF CONTENTS

Introduction

Thank you for purchasing this resource! You have made the choice to prepare yourself for a test that could have a huge impact on your future, and this guide is designed to help you be fully ready for test day. Obviously, it's important to have a solid understanding of the test material, but you also need to be prepared for the unique environment and stressors of the test, so that you can perform to the best of your abilities.

For this purpose, the first section that appears in this guide is the **Secret Keys**. We've devoted countless hours to meticulously researching what works and what doesn't, and we've boiled down our findings to the five most impactful steps you can take to improve your performance on the test. We start at the beginning with study planning and move through the preparation process, all the way to the testing strategies that will help you get the most out of what you know when you're finally sitting in front of the test.

We recommend that you start preparing for your test as far in advance as possible. However, if you've bought this guide as a last-minute study resource and only have a few days before your test, we recommend that you skip over the first two Secret Keys since they address a long-term study plan.

If you struggle with **test anxiety**, we strongly encourage you to check out our recommendations for how you can overcome it. Test anxiety is a formidable foe, but it can be beaten, and we want to make sure you have the tools you need to defeat it.

Review Video Directory

As you work your way through this guide, you will see numerous review video links interspersed with the written content. If you would like to access all of these review videos in one place, click on the video directory link found on the bonus page: **mometrix.com/bonus948/emt**

SCAN HERE

Secret Key #1 – Plan Big, Study Small

There's a lot riding on your performance. If you want to ace this test, you're going to need to keep your skills sharp and the material fresh in your mind. You need a plan that lets you review everything you need to know while still fitting in your schedule. We'll break this strategy down into three categories.

Information Organization

Start with the information you already have: the official test outline. From this, you can make a complete list of all the concepts you need to cover before the test. Organize these concepts into groups that can be studied together, and create a list of any related vocabulary you need to learn so you can brush up on any difficult terms. You'll want to keep this vocabulary list handy once you actually start studying since you may need to add to it along the way.

Time Management

Once you have your set of study concepts, decide how to spread them out over the time you have left before the test. Break your study plan into small, clear goals so you have a manageable task for each day and know exactly what you're doing. Then just focus on one small step at a time. When you manage your time this way, you don't need to spend hours at a time studying. Studying a small block of content for a short period each day helps you retain information better and avoid stressing over how much you have left to do. You can relax knowing that you have a plan to cover everything in time. In order for this strategy to be effective though, you have to start studying early and stick to your schedule. Avoid the exhaustion and futility that comes from last-minute cramming!

Study Environment

The environment you study in has a big impact on your learning. Studying in a coffee shop, while probably more enjoyable, is not likely to be as fruitful as studying in a quiet room. It's important to keep distractions to a minimum. You're only planning to study for a short block of time, so make the most of it. Don't pause to check your phone or get up to find a snack. It's also important to **avoid multitasking**. Research has consistently shown that multitasking will make your studying dramatically less effective. Your study area should also be comfortable and well-lit so you don't have the distraction of straining your eyes or sitting on an uncomfortable chair.

 The time of day you study is also important. You want to be rested and alert. Don't wait until just before bedtime. Study when you'll be most likely to comprehend and remember. Even better, if you know what time of day your test will be, set that time aside for study. That way your brain will be used to working on that subject at that specific time and you'll have a better chance of recalling information.

Finally, it can be helpful to team up with others who are studying for the same test. Your actual studying should be done in as isolated an environment as possible, but the work of organizing the information and setting up the study plan can be divided up. In between study sessions, you can discuss with your teammates the concepts that you're all studying and quiz each other on the details. Just be sure that your teammates are as serious about the test as you are. If you find that your study time is being replaced with social time, you might need to find a new team.

2

Secret Key #2 – Make Your Studying Count

You're devoting a lot of time and effort to preparing for this test, so you want to be absolutely certain it will pay off. This means doing more than just reading the content and hoping you can remember it on test day. It's important to make every minute of study count. There are two main areas you can focus on to make your studying count.

Retention

It doesn't matter how much time you study if you can't remember the material. You need to make sure you are retaining the concepts. To check your retention of the information you're learning, try recalling it at later times with minimal prompting. Try carrying around flashcards and glance at one or two from time to time or ask a friend who's also studying for the test to quiz you.

To enhance your retention, look for ways to put the information into practice so that you can apply it rather than simply recalling it. If you're using the information in practical ways, it will be much easier to remember. Similarly, it helps to solidify a concept in your mind if you're not only reading it to yourself but also explaining it to someone else. Ask a friend to let you teach them about a concept you're a little shaky on (or speak aloud to an imaginary audience if necessary). As you try to summarize, define, give examples, and answer your friend's questions, you'll understand the concepts better and they will stay with you longer. Finally, step back for a big picture view and ask yourself how each piece of information fits with the whole subject. When you link the different concepts together and see them working together as a whole, it's easier to remember the individual components.

Finally, practice showing your work on any multi-step problems, even if you're just studying. Writing out each step you take to solve a problem will help solidify the process in your mind, and you'll be more likely to remember it during the test.

Modality

Modality simply refers to the means or method by which you study. Choosing a study modality that fits your own individual learning style is crucial. No two people learn best in exactly the same way, so it's important to know your strengths and use them to your advantage.

For example, if you learn best by visualization, focus on visualizing a concept in your mind and draw an image or a diagram. Try color-coding your notes, illustrating them, or creating symbols that will trigger your mind to recall a learned concept. If you learn best by hearing or discussing information, find a study partner who learns the same way or read aloud to yourself. Think about how to put the information in your own words. Imagine that you are giving a lecture on the topic and record yourself so you can listen to it later.

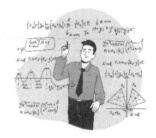

For any learning style, flashcards can be helpful. Organize the information so you can take advantage of spare moments to review. Underline key words or phrases. Use different colors for different categories. Mnemonic devices (such as creating a short list in which every item starts with the same letter) can also help with retention. Find what works best for you and use it to store the information in your mind most effectively and easily.

Secret Key #3 – Practice the Right Way

Your success on test day depends not only on how many hours you put into preparing, but also on whether you prepared the right way. It's good to check along the way to see if your studying is paying off. One of the most effective ways to do this is by taking practice tests to evaluate your progress. Practice tests are useful because they show exactly where you need to improve. Every time you take a practice test, pay special attention to these three groups of questions:

- The questions you got wrong
- The questions you had to guess on, even if you guessed right
- The questions you found difficult or slow to work through

This will show you exactly what your weak areas are, and where you need to devote more study time. Ask yourself why each of these questions gave you trouble. Was it because you didn't understand the material? Was it because you didn't remember the vocabulary? Do you need more repetitions on this type of question to build speed and confidence? Dig into those questions and figure out how you can strengthen your weak areas as you go back to review the material.

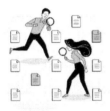 Additionally, many practice tests have a section explaining the answer choices. It can be tempting to read the explanation and think that you now have a good understanding of the concept. However, an explanation likely only covers part of the question's broader context. Even if the explanation makes perfect sense, **go back and investigate** every concept related to the question until you're positive you have a thorough understanding.

As you go along, keep in mind that the practice test is just that: practice. Memorizing these questions and answers will not be very helpful on the actual test because it is unlikely to have any of the same exact questions. If you only know the right answers to the sample questions, you won't be prepared for the real thing. **Study the concepts** until you understand them fully, and then you'll be able to answer any question that shows up on the test.

It's important to wait on the practice tests until you're ready. If you take a test on your first day of study, you may be overwhelmed by the amount of material covered and how much you need to learn. Work up to it gradually.

On test day, you'll need to be prepared for answering questions, managing your time, and using the test-taking strategies you've learned. It's a lot to balance, like a mental marathon that will have a big impact on your future. Like training for a marathon, you'll need to start slowly and work your way up. When test day arrives, you'll be ready.

Start with the strategies you've read in the first two Secret Keys—plan your course and study in the way that works best for you. If you have time, consider using multiple study resources to get different approaches to the same concepts. It can be helpful to see difficult concepts from more than one angle. Then find a good source for practice tests. Many times, the test website will suggest potential study resources or provide sample tests.

Practice Test Strategy

If you're able to find at least three practice tests, we recommend this strategy:

UNTIMED AND OPEN-BOOK PRACTICE

Take the first test with no time constraints and with your notes and study guide handy. Take your time and focus on applying the strategies you've learned.

TIMED AND OPEN-BOOK PRACTICE

Take the second practice test open-book as well, but set a timer and practice pacing yourself to finish in time.

TIMED AND CLOSED-BOOK PRACTICE

Take any other practice tests as if it were test day. Set a timer and put away your study materials. Sit at a table or desk in a quiet room, imagine yourself at the testing center, and answer questions as quickly and accurately as possible.

Keep repeating timed and closed-book tests on a regular basis until you run out of practice tests or it's time for the actual test. Your mind will be ready for the schedule and stress of test day, and you'll be able to focus on recalling the material you've learned.

Secret Key #4 – Pace Yourself

Once you're fully prepared for the material on the test, your biggest challenge on test day will be managing your time. Just knowing that the clock is ticking can make you panic even if you have plenty of time left. Work on pacing yourself so you can build confidence against the time constraints of the exam. Pacing is a difficult skill to master, especially in a high-pressure environment, so **practice is vital**.

Set time expectations for your pace based on how much time is available. For example, if a section has 60 questions and the time limit is 30 minutes, you know you have to average 30 seconds or less per question in order to answer them all. Although 30 seconds is the hard limit, set 25 seconds per question as your goal, so you reserve extra time to spend on harder questions. When you budget extra time for the harder questions, you no longer have any reason to stress when those questions take longer to answer.

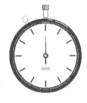

Don't let this time expectation distract you from working through the test at a calm, steady pace, but keep it in mind so you don't spend too much time on any one question. Recognize that taking extra time on one question you don't understand may keep you from answering two that you do understand later in the test. If your time limit for a question is up and you're still not sure of the answer, mark it and move on, and come back to it later if the time and the test format allow. If the testing format doesn't allow you to return to earlier questions, just make an educated guess; then put it out of your mind and move on.

On the easier questions, be careful not to rush. It may seem wise to hurry through them so you have more time for the challenging ones, but it's not worth missing one if you know the concept and just didn't take the time to read the question fully. Work efficiently but make sure you understand the question and have looked at all of the answer choices, since more than one may seem right at first.

Even if you're paying attention to the time, you may find yourself a little behind at some point. You should speed up to get back on track, but do so wisely. Don't panic; just take a few seconds less on each question until you're caught up. Don't guess without thinking, but do look through the answer choices and eliminate any you know are wrong. If you can get down to two choices, it is often worthwhile to guess from those. Once you've chosen an answer, move on and don't dwell on any that you skipped or had to hurry through. If a question was taking too long, chances are it was one of the harder ones, so you weren't as likely to get it right anyway.

On the other hand, if you find yourself getting ahead of schedule, it may be beneficial to slow down a little. The more quickly you work, the more likely you are to make a careless mistake that will affect your score. You've budgeted time for each question, so don't be afraid to spend that time. Practice an efficient but careful pace to get the most out of the time you have.

Secret Key #5 – Have a Plan for Guessing

When you're taking the test, you may find yourself stuck on a question. Some of the answer choices seem better than others, but you don't see the one answer choice that is obviously correct. What do you do?

The scenario described above is very common, yet most test takers have not effectively prepared for it. Developing and practicing a plan for guessing may be one of the single most effective uses of your time as you get ready for the exam.

In developing your plan for guessing, there are three questions to address:

- When should you start the guessing process?
- How should you narrow down the choices?
- Which answer should you choose?

When to Start the Guessing Process

Unless your plan for guessing is to select C every time (which, despite its merits, is not what we recommend), you need to leave yourself enough time to apply your answer elimination strategies. Since you have a limited amount of time for each question, that means that if you're going to give yourself the best shot at guessing correctly, you have to decide quickly whether or not you will guess.

Of course, the best-case scenario is that you don't have to guess at all, so first, see if you can answer the question based on your knowledge of the subject and basic reasoning skills. Focus on the key words in the question and try to jog your memory of related topics. Give yourself a chance to bring the knowledge to mind, but once you realize that you don't have (or you can't access) the knowledge you need to answer the question, it's time to start the guessing process.

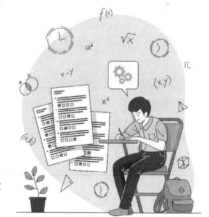

It's almost always better to start the guessing process too early than too late. It only takes a few seconds to remember something and answer the question from knowledge. Carefully eliminating wrong answer choices takes longer. Plus, going through the process of eliminating answer choices can actually help jog your memory.

Summary: Start the guessing process as soon as you decide that you can't answer the question based on your knowledge.

7

How to Narrow Down the Choices

The next chapter in this book (**Test-Taking Strategies**) includes a wide range of strategies for how to approach questions and how to look for answer choices to eliminate. You will definitely want to read those carefully, practice them, and figure out which ones work best for you. Here though, we're going to address a mindset rather than a particular strategy.

Your odds of guessing an answer correctly depend on how many options you are choosing from.

Number of options left	5	4	3	2	1
Odds of guessing correctly	20%	25%	33%	50%	100%

You can see from this chart just how valuable it is to be able to eliminate incorrect answers and make an educated guess, but there are two things that many test takers do that cause them to miss out on the benefits of guessing:

- Accidentally eliminating the correct answer
- Selecting an answer based on an impression

We'll look at the first one here, and the second one in the next section.

To avoid accidentally eliminating the correct answer, we recommend a thought exercise called **the $5 challenge**. In this challenge, you only eliminate an answer choice from contention if you are willing to bet $5 on it being wrong. Why $5? Five dollars is a small but not insignificant amount of money. It's an amount you could afford to lose but wouldn't want to throw away. And while losing

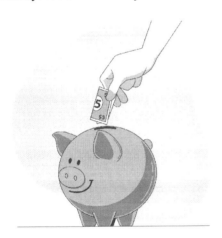

$5 once might not hurt too much, doing it twenty times will set you back $100. In the same way, each small decision you make—eliminating a choice here, guessing on a question there—won't by itself impact your score very much, but when you put them all together, they can make a big difference. By holding each answer choice elimination decision to a higher standard, you can reduce the risk of accidentally eliminating the correct answer.

The $5 challenge can also be applied in a positive sense: If you are willing to bet $5 that an answer choice *is* correct, go ahead and mark it as correct.

Summary: Only eliminate an answer choice if you are willing to bet $5 that it is wrong.

Which Answer to Choose

You're taking the test. You've run into a hard question and decided you'll have to guess. You've eliminated all the answer choices you're willing to bet $5 on. Now you have to pick an answer. Why do we even need to talk about this? Why can't you just pick whichever one you feel like when the time comes?

The answer to these questions is that if you don't come into the test with a plan, you'll rely on your impression to select an answer choice, and if you do that, you risk falling into a trap. The test writers know that everyone who takes their test will be guessing on some of the questions, so they intentionally write wrong answer choices to seem plausible. You still have to pick an answer though, and if the wrong answer choices are designed to look right, how can you ever be sure that you're not falling for their trap? The best solution we've found to this dilemma is to take the decision out of your hands entirely. Here is the process we recommend:

Once you've eliminated any choices that you are confident (willing to bet $5) are wrong, select the first remaining choice as your answer.

Whether you choose to select the first remaining choice, the second, or the last, the important thing is that you use some preselected standard. Using this approach guarantees that you will not be enticed into selecting an answer choice that looks right, because you are not basing your decision on how the answer choices look.

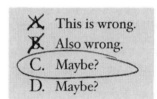

This is not meant to make you question your knowledge. Instead, it is to help you recognize the difference between your knowledge and your impressions. There's a huge difference between thinking an answer is right because of what you know, and thinking an answer is right because it looks or sounds like it should be right.

Summary: To ensure that your selection is appropriately random, make a predetermined selection from among all answer choices you have not eliminated.

Test-Taking Strategies

This section contains a list of test-taking strategies that you may find helpful as you work through the test. By taking what you know and applying logical thought, you can maximize your chances of answering any question correctly!

It is very important to realize that every question is different and every person is different: no single strategy will work on every question, and no single strategy will work for every person. That's why we've included all of them here, so you can try them out and determine which ones work best for different types of questions and which ones work best for you.

Question Strategies

⦿ READ CAREFULLY

Read the question and the answer choices carefully. Don't miss the question because you misread the terms. You have plenty of time to read each question thoroughly and make sure you understand what is being asked. Yet a happy medium must be attained, so don't waste too much time. You must read carefully and efficiently.

⦿ CONTEXTUAL CLUES

Look for contextual clues. If the question includes a word you are not familiar with, look at the immediate context for some indication of what the word might mean. Contextual clues can often give you all the information you need to decipher the meaning of an unfamiliar word. Even if you can't determine the meaning, you may be able to narrow down the possibilities enough to make a solid guess at the answer to the question.

⦿ PREFIXES

If you're having trouble with a word in the question or answer choices, try dissecting it. Take advantage of every clue that the word might include. Prefixes can be a huge help. Usually, they allow you to determine a basic meaning. *Pre-* means before, *post-* means after, *pro-* is positive, *de-* is negative. From prefixes, you can get an idea of the general meaning of the word and try to put it into context.

⦿ HEDGE WORDS

Watch out for critical hedge words, such as *likely, may, can, sometimes, often, almost, mostly, usually, generally, rarely,* and *sometimes.* Question writers insert these hedge phrases to cover every possibility. Often an answer choice will be wrong simply because it leaves no room for exception. Be on guard for answer choices that have definitive words such as *exactly* and *always.*

⦿ SWITCHBACK WORDS

Stay alert for *switchbacks.* These are the words and phrases frequently used to alert you to shifts in thought. The most common switchback words are *but, although,* and *however.* Others include *nevertheless, on the other hand, even though, while, in spite of, despite,* and *regardless of.* Switchback words are important to catch because they can change the direction of the question or an answer choice.

10

⊘ Face Value

When in doubt, use common sense. Accept the situation in the problem at face value. Don't read too much into it. These problems will not require you to make wild assumptions. If you have to go beyond creativity and warp time or space in order to have an answer choice fit the question, then you should move on and consider the other answer choices. These are normal problems rooted in reality. The applicable relationship or explanation may not be readily apparent, but it is there for you to figure out. Use your common sense to interpret anything that isn't clear.

Answer Choice Strategies

⊘ Answer Selection

The most thorough way to pick an answer choice is to identify and eliminate wrong answers until only one is left, then confirm it is the correct answer. Sometimes an answer choice may immediately seem right, but be careful. The test writers will usually put more than one reasonable answer choice on each question, so take a second to read all of them and make sure that the other choices are not equally obvious. As long as you have time left, it is better to read every answer choice than to pick the first one that looks right without checking the others.

⊘ Answer Choice Families

An answer choice family consists of two (in rare cases, three) answer choices that are very similar in construction and cannot all be true at the same time. If you see two answer choices that are direct opposites or parallels, one of them is usually the correct answer. For instance, if one answer choice says that quantity x increases and another either says that quantity x decreases (opposite) or says that quantity y increases (parallel), then those answer choices would fall into the same family. An answer choice that doesn't match the construction of the answer choice family is more likely to be incorrect. Most questions will not have answer choice families, but when they do appear, you should be prepared to recognize them.

⊘ Eliminate Answers

Eliminate answer choices as soon as you realize they are wrong, but make sure you consider all possibilities. If you are eliminating answer choices and realize that the last one you are left with is also wrong, don't panic. Start over and consider each choice again. There may be something you missed the first time that you will realize on the second pass.

⊘ Avoid Fact Traps

Don't be distracted by an answer choice that is factually true but doesn't answer the question. You are looking for the choice that answers the question. Stay focused on what the question is asking for so you don't accidentally pick an answer that is true but incorrect. Always go back to the question and make sure the answer choice you've selected actually answers the question and is not merely a true statement.

⊘ Extreme Statements

In general, you should avoid answers that put forth extreme actions as standard practice or proclaim controversial ideas as established fact. An answer choice that states the "process should be used in certain situations, if..." is much more likely to be correct than one that states the "process should be discontinued completely." The first is a calm rational statement and doesn't even make a definitive, uncompromising stance, using a hedge word *if* to provide wiggle room, whereas the second choice is far more extreme.

11

⊘ Benchmark

As you read through the answer choices and you come across one that seems to answer the question well, mentally select that answer choice. This is not your final answer, but it's the one that will help you evaluate the other answer choices. The one that you selected is your benchmark or standard for judging each of the other answer choices. Every other answer choice must be compared to your benchmark. That choice is correct until proven otherwise by another answer choice beating it. If you find a better answer, then that one becomes your new benchmark. Once you've decided that no other choice answers the question as well as your benchmark, you have your final answer.

⊘ Predict the Answer

Before you even start looking at the answer choices, it is often best to try to predict the answer. When you come up with the answer on your own, it is easier to avoid distractions and traps because you will know exactly what to look for. The right answer choice is unlikely to be word-for-word what you came up with, but it should be a close match. Even if you are confident that you have the right answer, you should still take the time to read each option before moving on.

General Strategies

⊘ Tough Questions

If you are stumped on a problem or it appears too hard or too difficult, don't waste time. Move on! Remember though, if you can quickly check for obviously incorrect answer choices, your chances of guessing correctly are greatly improved. Before you completely give up, at least try to knock out a couple of possible answers. Eliminate what you can and then guess at the remaining answer choices before moving on.

⊘ Check Your Work

Since you will probably not know every term listed and the answer to every question, it is important that you get credit for the ones that you do know. Don't miss any questions through careless mistakes. If at all possible, try to take a second to look back over your answer selection and make sure you've selected the correct answer choice and haven't made a costly careless mistake (such as marking an answer choice that you didn't mean to mark). This quick double check should more than pay for itself in caught mistakes for the time it costs.

⊘ Pace Yourself

It's easy to be overwhelmed when you're looking at a page full of questions; your mind is confused and full of random thoughts, and the clock is ticking down faster than you would like. Calm down and maintain the pace that you have set for yourself. Especially as you get down to the last few minutes of the test, don't let the small numbers on the clock make you panic. As long as you are on track by monitoring your pace, you are guaranteed to have time for each question.

⊘ Don't Rush

It is very easy to make errors when you are in a hurry. Maintaining a fast pace in answering questions is pointless if it makes you miss questions that you would have gotten right otherwise. Test writers like to include distracting information and wrong answers that seem right. Taking a little extra time to avoid careless mistakes can make all the difference in your test score. Find a pace that allows you to be confident in the answers that you select.

⊘ Keep Moving

Panicking will not help you pass the test, so do your best to stay calm and keep moving. Taking deep breaths and going through the answer elimination steps you practiced can help to break through a stress barrier and keep your pace.

Final Notes

The combination of a solid foundation of content knowledge and the confidence that comes from practicing your plan for applying that knowledge is the key to maximizing your performance on test day. As your foundation of content knowledge is built up and strengthened, you'll find that the strategies included in this chapter become more and more effective in helping you quickly sift through the distractions and traps of the test to isolate the correct answer.

Now that you're preparing to move forward into the test content chapters of this book, be sure to keep your goal in mind. As you read, think about how you will be able to apply this information on the test. If you've already seen sample questions for the test and you have an idea of the question format and style, try to come up with questions of your own that you can answer based on what you're reading. This will give you valuable practice applying your knowledge in the same ways you can expect to on test day.

Good luck and good studying!

A Note About EMT Interventions

Each EMS certification level has a specific scope of practice that dictates which interventions a certification holder may perform in the course of their job. An individual with an EMR certification is not permitted to perform all of the same interventions that an individual with an EMT certification may. Similarly, an Advanced EMT certification authorizes an individual to perform interventions that neither an EMT nor an EMR certification would allow.

As you read through this study guide, you will notice that we frequently provide information about all of the interventions that may be performed for a given emergency, not just those that are appropriate for this level of certification. Even though you may not be authorized to perform all of these interventions, we believe it will be helpful for you to be aware that they exist, as you may find yourself working with others in the EMS community with a higher level of certification, and knowing about what they are permitted to do may help you respond more effectively in a given situation. **You should never attempt to perform any intervention that is outside the scope of practice for your certification.**

As you continue your journey toward certification, we at Mometrix applaud you for your desire to serve your community in this way. Best of luck in your studying!

Foundational Knowledge and Skills

Medical Terminology

BODY PLANES AND ANATOMIC TERMS

Body planes include the following:

- **Sagittal/Lateral**: Vertical plane separating right from left
- **Median/Midsagittal**: Sagittal plane at the midline (middle) separating the body into equal halves
- **Coronal/Frontal**: Vertical plane separating anterior (front) from posterior (back)
- **Axial/Transverse**: Horizontal plane that separates the body into superior (upper) and inferior (lower) parts

A **cross section** is an axial/transverse (horizontal) cut through a tissue specimen or body structure, whereas a **longitudinal section** is a sagittal or coronal (vertical) cut. **Medial** is toward the midline, whereas **lateral** is away from the midline and to the side. **Distal** is farther from the point of reference, and **proximal** is closer. When describing an area of the patient's body, the description should be patient oriented, using phrases such as "patient's left" and "patient's right" to ensure accurate interpretation.

Body planes and anatomic terms

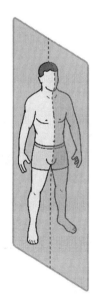 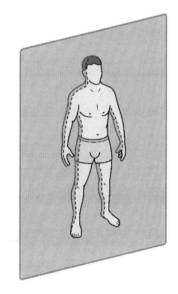 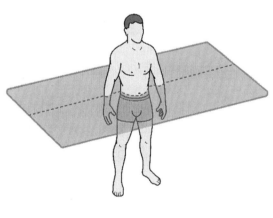

Sagittal/Lateral   Coronal/Frontal   Axial/Transverse

COMMON MEDICAL PREFIXES

Term	Meaning	Examples
Cardio-	Heart	Cardiovascular (heart and vessels), cardiology (study of the heart)
Neuro-	Nerves	Neurology (study of the nerves), neuron (nerve cell)
Hyper-	Enlarged, excessive, high	Hypertrophy (enlarged tissue), hyperemesis (excessive vomiting), hyperactive (overactive), hypertension (high BP)
Hypo-	Under, beneath, low	Hypoglycemia (low blood sugar), hypotension (low BP), hypoxia (low oxygen)
Naso-	Nose	Nasopharyngeal (nose and throat), nasal (referring to the nose)
Oro-	Mouth	Oropharyngeal (mouth and throat), oral (referring to the mouth)
Arterio-	Artery	Arteriovenous (artery and vein), arterial (referring to arteries)
Hemo- Hemato-	Blood	Hemolysis (breakdown of blood), hemoglobin (blood component), hematology (study of blood)
Therm-	Temperature	Thermoregulation (temperature regulation), thermometer (temperature measurement)
Vaso-	Vessels	Vasoconstriction (narrowing of vessels), vasodilation (widening of vessels)
Tachy-	Rapid	Tachycardia (rapid heart rate), tachypnea (rapid respirations)
Brady-	Slow	Bradycardia (slow heart rate), bradypnea (slow respirations)

Pharmacology

FIVE RIGHTS OF MEDICATION ADMINISTRATION

The EMS provider may assist patients to self-administer medications or administer them directly depending on the scope of practice and protocols. Medical direction may be offline, which means standing orders are available to treat specific conditions or written protocols have been established that must be followed. Online medical direction requires verbal contact with a medical director. When receiving an online medication order, the EMS provider should use the echo (read-back) technique (repeating back the orders to ensure that they were understood correctly) and clarify any orders that are confusing or unclear.

The **five rights of medication administration** include the following:

1. **Right patient**: Prescribed specifically for that patient
2. **Right medication**: Correct choice for the patient's condition and matches the prescription
3. **Right route**: Appropriate for the patient's condition, enteral or parenteral
4. **Right dose**: As prescribed and appropriate for the patient's age, weight, and condition
5. **Right time**: Medication not expired, is administered at the time ordered (e.g., "stat" (immediately) or "every 5 minutes × 3")

> **Review Video: Top 5 Pharmacology Review Mnemonics**
> Visit mometrix.com/academy and enter code: 119193

NALOXONE FOR OPIOID OVERDOSE

Naloxone (Narcan) autoinjector contains a single dose of 2 mg naloxone in 0.4 mL solution and is delivered IM or SQ only. Naloxone autoinjector is used to treat suspected opioid overdose in adult and pediatric patients. Opioid overdose is characterized by lethargy, respiratory depression, sleepiness, pinpoint pupils, confusion, and non-responsiveness. The label contains printed directions, and the electronic voice instruction system guides the user as well. Procedure:

1. Remove red safety guard.
2. Administer into the anterolateral aspect of the thigh. May be administered through clothing if necessary. For infants under one year, pinch the thigh muscle before administering the medication.
3. Injections may be repeated every 2-3 minutes as needed with new devices.

Naloxone (Narcan) 4 mg nasal spray is used to treat opioid overdose in adults and pediatric patients. Procedure:

1. Open container and remove the device.
2. Place thumb on the plunger and 2 fingers on the nozzle.
3. Place the tip of the nozzle into one of the patient's nostrils until the fingers contact the patient's nose.
4. Depress the plunger. Additional doses may be given every 2-3 minutes using a new device each time.

AUTOINJECTORS FOR NERVE AGENT EXPOSURE

Autoinjectors are spring-loaded syringe/needle devices that contain preloaded doses of medication and can be easily administered by following the directions on the devices. Autoinjectors are available for nerve agent treatment for emergency medical personnel—Mark I and DuoDote.

- **Atropine autoinjector**: For symptoms of nerve damage (increases heart rate, dries secretions, dilates pupils, and reduces GI upset)
- **Pralidoxime (2-PAM chloride) autoinjector**: For symptoms of nerve damage, twitching, and difficulty breathing
- **Diazepam autoinjector**: For convulsions associated with nerve agents

Wear appropriate PPE, remove the safety cap, cleanse the skin with alcohol, and (holding the device perpendicular to the skin) apply firm pressure with the tip of the injector against the skin in the outer thigh until the device fires the needle into the muscle tissue (avoid jabbing). Then, hold the autoinjector in place for at least 10 seconds to ensure that the medication is completely injected. Carefully remove the needle from the skin. Avoid touching the needle, and do not attempt to recap it. Dispose of the intact device in a sharps container.

NEBULIZED, INHALED AND SUBLINGUAL ROUTES OF MEDICATION ADMINISTRATION

Nebulized medications are delivered with compressed air or high flow oxygen (6-8 L/min) to aerosolize the small volume of liquid into a mist. The patient breathes the aerosolized medication through a mouthpiece or a securely fitted mask. Nebulized medications, such as albuterol and steroids, are often given to patients with respiratory diseases, such as asthma and COPD. Nebulizers are often easier for patients to use than **inhaled medications** per a metered-dose-inhalers, especially if they are at all confused. Inhaled medications are provided per a metered-dose inhaler (MDI) that delivers a specific dose of aerosolized medication, but the patient must be able to coordinate breathing with the dose (puff) and to hold her breath for 10 seconds after delivery of the drug. For both nebulized and inhaled medications, patients should sit upright.

Mucosal/sublingual/buccal medications are usually provided in thin wafers that dissolve on contact with saliva. Sublingual medications are placed under the tongue and mucosal/buccal medications between the gums and the cheek. The medications are absorbed quickly into the bloodstream so dosage is often lower than other routes. Eating, drinking fluids, and smoking can affect absorption of the drugs.

Metered-Dose Inhaler (MIDI/MDI) and the Small-Volume Nebulizer

The EMT may administer or assist the patient with use of a metered-dose inhaler (MIDI/MDI) or a small-volume nebulizer for medications such as albuterol, according to protocol, as follows:

- The **MIDI/MDI** is a pressurized cartridge that is used for the administration of a specific dose of an aerosolized medication. Shake the medication vigorously before use, prime if it is the initial use, position 4 cm (two finger widths) away from the patient's mouth or between the lips, have the patient exhale and breathe in slowly and completely while the MIDI is activated, and then have the patient hold his breath for 10 seconds, waiting 1 minute between puffs. Stop the treatment if the patient becomes shaky, dizzy, coughs uncontrollably, has palpitations, or has a pulse increase of ≥20 bpm. Resume slowly after 5-10 minutes.
- A **small-volume nebulizer** includes a nebulizer cup that holds 2-4 mL of medication, air tubing, a compressor to aerosolize the medication, and a T-piece and mouthpiece or face mask for delivery. Dilute the medication with sterile water or NS, not tap water, if necessary. Have the patient sit upright for treatment, breathing normally through the mouth, using the mouthpiece or face mask.

Commonly Administered Medications by the EMT

Medication	Dose/Route/Use	Side effects/Interactions
Aspirin	Orally, 325 mg, chew and swallow for fast action when having a heart attack.	Avoid with signs of stroke or gastrointestinal (GI) bleeding. Decreases clotting time and may increase the risk of bleeding.
Glucose	Orally for hypoglycemia. May be in liquid or tablet form, or a glass of orange juice may be given.	Minimal unless hyperglycemic.
Oxygen	Inhaled; usually 2-6 L, but it varies according to protocol.	Minimal, although oxygen toxicity can occur with high doses for prolonged periods of time.
Bronchodilators (albuterol, levalbuterol)	Inhaled; usually two puffs of a handheld inhaler. Dosage varies according to the medication. Used for bronchospasm, wheezing.	Adverse effects: tachycardia, dizziness, nervousness, tremor, headache, rhinitis, increased cough.
Epinephrine (EpiPen)	Autoinjector; 0.3 mg at 1:1000 for ≥66 lb, 0.15 mg at 1:2000 for 33-66 lb for severe allergic reaction/anaphylaxis.	Avoid using with antihistamines, thyroid hormones, and alpha blockers. Adverse effects: drowsiness, headache, palpitations, nervousness, tremors.
Nitroglycerin	Sublingually for angina (chest pain); 0.3-0.6 mg, repeated every 5 minutes up to 3 times.	Avoid with myocardial infarction. Adverse effects: headache, flushing, dizziness, orthostatic hypotension, palpitations. Interactions: Avoid with erectile dysfunction drugs (sildenafil, tadalafil, vardenafil).

EMT Assessment

PRIMARY ASSESSMENT

After surveying the environment for safety issues, the EMS provider should quickly conduct a **primary assessment** to identify conditions that are life-threatening, as follows:

- **Level of consciousness**: Alert, responsive to verbal stimuli, responsive to painful stimuli, nonresponsive
- **Breathing status**: Normal, abnormal, rate abnormalities (>24 or <8), apnea, choking, normal or abnormal chest movement, chest rise and fall, noisy respirations, use of accessory muscles, tripod position, nasal flaring
- **Circulatory status**: Radial, carotid pulse, pulse abnormalities, major bleeding, skin color (pink, blue [cyanotic], pale), skin temperature, skin moisture, capillary refill, signs of shock

Life-threatening conditions must be treated immediately, as follows:

- Carotid pulse present with no radial pulse: Lay the patient flat and elevate his or her feet 8-12 inches.
- No pulse: Begin CPR.
- Shock: Lay the patient flat, elevate his or her feet 8-12 inches, and administer oxygen at 15 L/min.
- Bleeding: Apply pressure to control any bleeding.
- Abnormal breathing: Provide oxygen with a nonrebreather mask. If the patient is unresponsive, cyanotic, or in respiratory distress, use a BVM with supplemental oxygen.
- Unresponsive: Ensure a patent airway.

Based on the assessment, the patient is classified as stable, potentially unstable, or unstable.

HISTORY TAKING ON ARRIVAL AT A SCENE

History taking should include the following:

- **Chief complaint**: If the patient is unable to explain, information may be gathered from his or her family, friends, or others who are present. Look for a medical alert bracelet or other such jewelry.
- **Nature of the illness or mechanism of injury**: Reason for calling EMS, cause of injury, type of illness. Look for environmental clues (fire, drug paraphernalia, motor vehicle accident).
- **Signs and symptoms observed or reported by the patient**: Skin temperature, open wounds, BP abnormalities, pain, or difficulty breathing.
- **Precipitating events**: Falls, accidents, violence, eating, exercising, walking, driving.
- **Pediatric considerations**: Check capillary refill to assess blood flow in infants and children younger than 6. Assess the pulse at the brachial artery (inside of the upper arm) for infants up to 1 year of age and the carotid artery in the neck for children older than 1 year. May need to use distraction to gain trust and alleviate fear. Encourage the parents/caregivers to hold the child if possible and assist in calming the child.
- **Geriatric (older adult) considerations**: Determine if the patient needs assistive devices, such as hearing aids, eyeglasses, cane, walker, or dentures.

OPQRST METHOD OF HISTORY TAKING

O	Onset	The time that the symptoms associated with this event started.
P	Provocative; palliative. Positioning	That which makes it better; that which makes it worse. The position that the patient is in on arrival and the need to remain in this position or to move him or her.
Q	Quality of discomfort	Burning, stabbing, nagging, crushing, sharp, or dull.
R	Radiation of pain	Area to which the pain moves from the original site.
S	Severity of pain	Based on a 1-to-10 or other appropriate scale.
T	Time	Historical onset, such as earlier, similar events.

SAMPLE METHOD OF HISTORY TAKING

S	Signs and symptoms	Pain, bleeding, shortness of breath, injuries, fever, rash.
A	Allergies	Medications, environmental (foods, insects, plants, animals).
M	Medications	Prescribed, over-the-counter (OTC) vitamins/minerals, birth control and erectile dysfunction medications, herbal preparations, recreational drugs, other people's medications.
P	Past pertinent history	Especially related to the current event.
L	Last oral intake	Foods, fluids, other substances.
E	Events (precipitating)	Occurrence just prior to event.

TAKING A HISTORY OF SENSITIVE TOPICS

When asking a patient about **sensitive topics,** the EMS provider should try to provide as much privacy as possible in an emergent situation in order to maintain confidentiality and protect the patient from reprisals. The EMS provider should ask questions directly in a straightforward and nonjudgmental manner, stressing the need for information in order to help the patient, especially if the patient is reluctant to answer. Sensitive topics include the following:

- **Sexual history**: People who engage in unusual or unhealthy sexual practices, such as sadomasochism, autoerotic asphyxiation, swinging, and prostitution, are often reluctant to admit to those practices. Adolescents may be especially reluctant to admit they are pregnant or have engaged in sexual activity or have had an abortion. Males (especially those older than age 40) should be asked about the use of erectile dysfunction drugs (such as Viagra) because they are a contraindication to some medical treatments.
- **Physical/Sexual abuse and/or violence**: Victims often lie about abuse to defend the abuser or out of shame or fear of further violence.
- **Alcohol/Drug use and abuse**: Patients often underreport the extent of their drinking or drug taking or deny it altogether. Patients may be concerned about legal actions, such as if they have been driving drunk and gotten into an accident.

SPECIAL HISTORY-TAKING CHALLENGES

Special history-taking challenges include the following:

- **Silent patient**: Be patient, sensitive, and alert for nonverbal clues.
- **Talkative patient**: Allow the patient to speak freely for a few minutes and then periodically summarize.
- **Anxious patient**: Be patient, provide reassurance, and explain all procedures.
- **Patient with multiple complaints**: Ask the patient to help prioritize his or her issues.
- **Hostile/angry patient**: Remain calm; respond as appropriate.
- **Intoxicated patient**: Avoid cornering, belittling, or challenging the patient or asking the patient to lower his or her voice or stop swearing. Remain calm and treat the patient with respect.
- **Depressed, crying patient**: Question the severity of the patient's depression; listen and remain supportive and nonjudgmental.
- **Patient with a language barrier**: Use a translator if possible. Use hand gestures. Show the equipment before using it; point to the part of the body where the equipment will be used.
- **Patient with a visual impairment**: Announce one's presence and explain all procedures verbally. Tell the patient before touching him or her.
- **Patient with a hearing impairment**: Determine if the patient has a hearing aid, and obtain it if possible. Speak slowly and clearly, facing the patient for any hearing deficit. If the patient has no hearing, use writing, hand gestures, and demonstrations to communicate.

SECONDARY ASSESSMENT

Following completion of the primary assessment and after attending to any life-threatening problems that are identified, carry out a **secondary assessment** as follows:

- **Measure vital signs**: Pulse (radial to carotid for adults and brachial for infants and small children), respiration rate, and BP. Using the correct BP cuff size is essential for accuracy. The length of the bladder in the cuff should be equal to 80% of the arm's circumference, and the lower edge of the cuff when positioned should end about one inch above the antecubital fossa (inner elbow). Inflate the cuff to 160-180 initially, and increase the pressure if pulse sounds are heard at that level.
- **Ask further questions as indicated**: These may focus on the primary complaint or others, depending on the situation.
- **Conduct a physical examination**: Examine the body; palpate for areas of tenderness or swelling; auscultate heart, lung, and abdominal sounds; and note any injuries. Do a brief head-to-toe assessment, and compare one side of the body with the other, noting any asymmetry.
- **Treat any life-threatening injuries or conditions** noted immediately.

REASSESSMENT

Reassessment involves ongoing monitoring of the patient at regular intervals to determine changes in his or her condition or trends such as decreasing BP or increasing agitation. **Reassessment** is done after a secondary assessment. Unstable patients should be reassessed at least every 5 minutes and stable patients every 15 minutes. Reassessment should include reviewing the primary assessment, taking vital signs, repeating the physical examination (including evaluation of mental status), and monitoring the chief complaint and response to interventions. Reassessment findings should be compared to baseline findings. The patient's airway, ventilation, and circulation should be reassessed as well as the patient's degree of pain—stable, better, or worse. Each intervention should be reassessed for effectiveness and the need for modifications of treatment or if new interventions should be determined. If the patient is receiving oxygen, the tank and all of the equipment should be checked to ensure that they are functioning properly.

NORMAL VITAL SIGNS FROM NEONATE TO LATE ADULTHOOD

Age	Heart rate	Respirations	BP (mmHg)
Neonate (0-12 mo.)	100–220 (average 140–160); slows after ~3 months	40–60 for a few minutes, then 30–40	Systolic 70–90
Toddler (12–36 mo.)	80–130	20–30	Systolic 70–100
Preschooler (3-5)	80–120	20–30	Systolic 80–110
School aged (6–12)	70–110	20–30	80–120/60–80
Adolescent (13–18)	55–100	12–20	110–131/64–84
Early adult (19–40)	60–100 (average 80)	12–20	100–119/60–79 to 140/90 (high)
Middle adult (41–60)	60–100 (average 80)	12–20	100–119/60–79 to 140/90 (high)
Late adult (61+)	60–100 (average 70)	12–20	100–119/60–79 to 140/90 (high)

ASSESSMENT OF FUNCTIONAL ABILITIES

Functional abilities should ideally be assessed in an active manner, with the person demonstrating the ability to sit; stand; get on and off of the toilet; walk; bend down; remove shoes, shirt, or jacket and then put them on again; listen; read; and answer questions. However, in an emergent situation, this type of assessment is often not possible. Careful questioning about the home environment can help with approximating the type of activities required and physical limitations that the patient experiences. A careful history of functional ability can pinpoint when and if changes occurred. Again, specific questioning guides patients: "When did you begin to use a cane?" "How old were you when you stopped using the tub?" "What is the biggest problem with caring for yourself?" or "When did you have a hip replacement, and how has that changed your life?"

INSTRUMENTAL ACTIVITIES OF DAILY LIVING (IADL) ASSESSMENT TOOL

Instrumental Activities of Daily Living (IADL) assessment tool measures eight activities necessary for an adult to function independently. This tool helps to determine the need for supportive services. Eight activities are each assigned as 0 (cannot do independently) or 1 (minimal or adequate degree of ability), so the total score ranges from 0 to 8, with a higher score indicating more independence in care. Abilities that are measured include the following:

1. Telephone use (ability to look up numbers and/or call numbers)
2. Shopping for food, clothes, or needed items
3. Food preparation (plans diet and prepares food)
4. Housekeeping (ability to perform all or part of household duties)
5. Laundry (can wash all or some of personal clothes and linen)
6. Transportation availability (ability to drive or use public transportation)
7. Medication (ability to be responsible for managing prescriptions and taking medications)
8. Financial responsibility (ability to keep track of finances, pay bills, and budget correctly)

Labs and Point of Care Testing

BLOOD GLUCOSE MONITORING

Blood glucose monitoring is done with a glucometer. Testing is indicated with a decreased level of consciousness or confusion in a diabetic patient or a decreased level of consciousness with the cause being unknown. The glucometer must be calibrated and tested regularly. Test results from capillary blood tend to be lower than test results on venous blood. The **testing procedure** is as follows:

- Wipe the site with an alcohol swab. The alcohol must be thoroughly dried before puncture, or it may interfere with the test results.
- Prick the side of the finger pad with a lancet or lancing device rather than the fingertip because the fingertip is more sensitive.
- Express a drop of blood onto the test strip.
- Insert the test strip into the glucometer according to the manufacturer's recommendations.
- Read the test results.
- Dispose of the lancet in a sharps container.

Warming the hand or lowering it may help to ensure adequate blood for the test. Hypoglycemia (low blood sugar/insulin reaction) is a reading of ≤70 mg/dL. Hyperglycemia (high blood sugar) is a reading of ≥160 mg/dL.

Airway, Respiration, and Ventilation

Airway, Respiration, and Ventilation Management

UPPER RESPIRATORY SYSTEM

Air enters the upper respiratory system through the **nasal cavity** and/or mouth, where it is warmed and moistened by **nasal and oral mucosa**. The four pairs of **paranasal sinuses** aid in warming and moistening the air (see graphic below). The air passes through the **pharynx**: **nasopharynx**, **oropharynx**, and **laryngopharynx/hypopharynx** (below and behind the larynx and epiglottis). Air passes behind or past the **soft palate** (the soft tissue at the back of the mouth) and the **uvula**, which hangs from the soft palate and into the lower respiratory system. The **hyoid bone** is above the Adam's apple and helps support the larynx. The **vallecula** ("spit trap") is at the root of the tongue. The **adenoids** (pharyngeal tonsils) are located on the posterior wall of the nasopharynx, and the **palatine tonsils** are on the back of the mouth on either side of the tongue. The adenoids and tonsils may become infected and swollen, obstructing the airway. The jawbones include the maxilla (upper) and mandible (lower). The jugular notch is the visible depression between the neck and clavicles (collarbones).

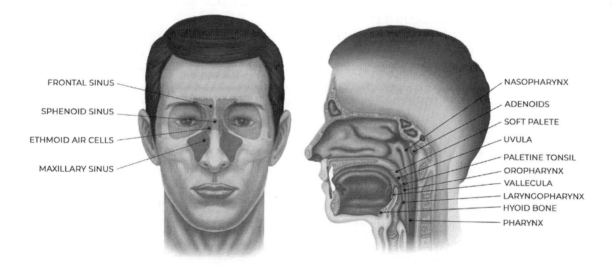

FRONTAL SINUS
SPHENOID SINUS
ETHMOID AIR CELLS
MAXILLARY SINUS

NASOPHARYNX
ADENOIDS
SOFT PALETE
UVULA
PALETINE TONSIL
OROPHARYNX
VALLECULA
LARYNGOPHARYNX
HYOID BONE
PHARYNX

> **Review Video: Respiratory System**
> Visit mometrix.com/academy and enter code: 783075

25

LOWER RESPIRATORY SYSTEM

Air passes from the upper respiratory system and the pharynx to the lower respiratory system and the **larynx** (voice box) into the **trachea** (windpipe). The **epiglottis** is a cartilage flap attached to the **thyroid cartilage** (above the cricoid cartilage), and it closes over the larynx and **glottis** (vocal cords) when swallowing, so food enters the esophagus. The trachea branches into two (right and left) **bronchi** that carry the air into the **lungs**. Each bronchus branches into smaller **bronchioles** and **alveoli** (small air sacs), which are connected to the ends of the bronchioles. The alveoli are covered with webs of tiny venous capillaries that deliver carbon dioxide and arterial capillaries that pick up oxygen. Muscles of respiration are the **diaphragm**, which is enervated by the **phrenic nerve**, and the **intercostal muscles**, but **accessory muscles** in the neck and collarbone area may help during respiratory distress.

PHYSIOLOGY OF RESPIRATION

The physiology of respiration includes the following:

1. **Ventilation**: Movement of air in and out of the lungs during inhalation and exhalation. Breathing may be impaired by disease (muscular dystrophy), drugs, trauma, bronchoconstriction, allergic reactions, foreign body obstructions, and infection.
2. **Oxygenation**: The process by which oxygen molecules bind to hemoglobin in the blood. The blood saturation level reflects the amount of oxygen that is dissolved in the blood and available to body tissues, and it should be ≥95%.
3. **Respiration**: The process by which the lungs exchange carbon dioxide for oxygen in the alveoli and provide this oxygenated blood to body tissues. Respiration may be external (inspiration, expiration), internal (exchange of gas), or cellular (cells perform tasks that require oxygen and glucose [sugar] and produce carbon dioxide as a waste product). Respiration may be impaired by a lack of air, toxins/poisons, and ineffective circulation (shock, cardiac arrest).

KEY ELEMENTS OF RESPIRATION

Key elements of respiration include the following:

- **Tidal volume**: Normal volume of gas inhaled during one respiration cycle (approximately 500 mL in a healthy adult, 6–8 mL/kg for children, and 5–7 mL/kg for neonates)
- **Inspiratory reserve volume**: Volume of air inhaled that is greater than the tidal volume during forced deep inhalation (up to 3000 mL)
- **Dead space**: Volume of inhaled gas that does not take part in gas exchange
- **Alveolar dead space**: Volume of alveoli that are ventilated but not perfused
- **Vital capacity**: Maximum volume of gas that can be forcefully exhaled from the lungs following a full inhalation
- **Minute volume**: Volume of gas expelled from the lungs in one minute (the respiratory rate × the tidal volume)
- **Residual volume**: Volume of gas remaining in the lungs after one full, forced exhalation
- **Total lung capacity**: Vital capacity plus residual volume; the total volume that the lungs can contain (usually about 6000 mL for adults)
- **Cellular respiration**: Use of oxygen and glucose to produce energy at the cellular level and the creation of water and carbon dioxide as by-products of metabolism

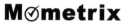

THE ROLE OF THE LUNGS IN EXTERNAL AND INTERNAL RESPIRATION

The lungs, located in the thoracic cavity and surrounded by pleural membranes, facilitate breathing through changes in pressure. When inhaling, the lungs and thoracic cavity expand, decreasing air pressure inside and forcing air from outside to enter. When exhaling, the pressure increases as the lungs and thoracic cavity contract, forcing air out of the lungs. The phrenic and intercostal nerves cause the diaphragm and intercostal muscles to contract and relax.

- **External respiration** occurs with gas exchange (oxygen for carbon dioxide) at the alveoli. The respiratory center in the brain (medulla oblongata) controls the breathing rate in response to chemoreceptors in the arteries that monitor levels of oxygen and carbon dioxide.
- **Internal respiration** occurs with gas exchange in the tissue cells. Physiologic dead spaces are those areas of the lung (including impaired alveoli) where gas exchange does not occur.

OXYGENATION AND PERFUSION IN THE LIFE SUPPORT CHAIN

Critical to the life support chain are oxygenation and perfusion. **Oxygenation** involves gas exchange of carbon dioxide for oxygen at the alveolar/capillary level and the cell/capillary level. **Perfusion** involves the transport of blood, which carries oxygen, glucose, and other nutrients as well as waste products throughout the body. Oxygen and glucose are essential for cell functioning. Glucose is produced by the digestion of carbohydrates (starches). Glucose is the primary energy source for the body, and its use is controlled by insulin, which is produced by the pancreas. Excess glucose is stored in the liver as glycogen for later use or is converted to fat. These fundamental elements are affected by the composition of ambient air (usually 21% oxygen), airway patency, ventilation, regulation of respiration, blood volume and transport, heart action, and blood vessel size and resistance.

PEDIATRIC AND OLDER ADULT AIRWAYS

Special **considerations** should be given to both pediatric and older adult airways:

- **Pediatric airways**: Infants are obligate nasal breathers for the first two to four months and usually only breathe through the nose, although they can generally breathe through the mouth if necessary. However, if nasal passages are blocked, they may quickly develop respiratory distress. Chest wall compliance is greater in infants and small children, so they must work harder than an adult to move the same amount of air. Additionally, proportionally the airway is smaller, the tongue is larger, and the cartilage is softer, increasing the risk of obstruction.
- **Older adult airways**: Breathing capacity tends to decline after age 40 because the number of alveoli decreases and the size of alveoli increases, resulting in less surface for, and less efficient, gas exchange. Lung elasticity also decreases, resulting in decreased vital capacity. The chest muscles tend to weaken and stiffen with age, and older adults have a lowered ability to cough and clear the airways.

AIRWAY ASSESSMENT AND MANUAL MEASURES TO CLEAR THE AIRWAY

Indications of an adequate airway include a normal voice and speaking ability and audible and visible air exchange. Indications of inadequate airway include unusual breathing sounds (wheezing, stridor), hoarse voice/inability to speak, and no audible or visible air exchange. Airway obstruction may result from the tongue falling back, food, a foreign body, vomit, blood, teeth, and edema (swelling). **Maneuvers** include the following:

- **Head tilt/chin lift**: Hyperextend the neck by tilting the patient's head back with one hand on his or her forehead to straighten the airway and lift the tongue. Then lift the chin and pull forward with the fingers of the other hand under the chin with the thumb on top. The chin lift pulls the mandible (jaw) forward. This prevents the tongue from blocking the pharynx. Contraindications to the head tilt/chin lift include suspected cervical spine and neck injuries.
- **Jaw thrust**: This technique is used with a suspected spinal cord or neck injury in which extending the neck must be avoided. From behind, place the fingers behind the angles of the patient's lower jaw and place your thumbs on the chin; move the jaw upward until it is extended while using the thumbs to slightly open the patient's mouth. Contraindications include severe facial injuries.
- **Modified chin lift/jaw thrust**: This technique is used with a suspected spinal cord/neck injury with an unstable cervical spine. From the head of the patient, place the thumbs on his or her cheekbones, place the fingers under the patient's mandible, and then pull the mandible upward with the fingers while applying pressure with the thumbs. If using a mask for ventilation, place the mask in position and secure it with the thumbs while the fingers thrust the patient's jaw forward.

ASSESSMENT OF OXYGENATION

Assessment of oxygenation includes the following:

1. **Evaluate respirations**: Note the signs of respiratory distress—rapid breathing, slow breathing, use of accessory muscles, nasal flaring, and sternal retraction—because they may indicate inadequate oxygenation.
2. **Assess mental status**: Confusion may be associated with hypo-oxygenation (low oxygen), but it's important to determine a baseline mental status if possible because the patient may have dementia or may be confused because of medications.
3. **Assess skin**: Note cyanosis (blue tinge) especially around the mouth, fingertips, and oral mucous membranes because this indicates a lack of oxygen. Another sign is pallor. Mottling of the skin, purplish or reddish discoloration especially on the knees and feet, indicates hypo-oxygenation and is a common indication that death is near.
4. **Monitor pulse oximetry**: Oxygen saturation should be 95%–100%. If a patient has mild respiratory disease, the pulse oximetry level may be as low as 90% and still be within the normal range for the patient. Readings of less than 90%–92% indicate hypoxemia (low oxygen in the blood).

ASSESSMENT OF RESPIRATIONS AND SUPPLEMENTAL OXYGEN ADMINISTRATION

When assessing respirations, the EMS provider should note the patient's gag reflex and rate of respirations (whether it is normal for the patient's age or too fast, too slow, or absent). The provider should also evaluate the rise and fall of the chest and any abnormal movements (such as sternal retraction, nasal flaring) noisy breathing (gurgling, wheezing), the use of accessory muscles, or the tripod position (sitting, leaning forward, and supporting the body with the hands).

If breathing is abnormal or the pulse oximetry is less than 95%, the EMS provider should take precautions against bloodstream infection (BSI) and administer **supplemental oxygen** with a **nonrebreather mask** with the oxygen set at 12–15 L. The reservoir bag of the mask must be completely filled before applying the mask to the patient, securing it with an elastic band about the head. If the patient cannot tolerate the nonrebreather mask, then a **nasal cannula** may be used with the oxygen flow set at 4–6 L, the prongs inserted into the nostrils, and tubing secured by looping over the ears and tightening under the chin.

ASSESSMENT OF VENTILATION

Ventilation is adequate if the respiratory rate, depth of respiration, and effort of breathing are normal. **Signs of inadequate ventilation** include the following:

1. **Increased effort of breathing**: Nasal flaring, sternal retraction (infants), use of abdominal or intercostal (between the ribs) muscles, sweating, sitting in the tripod position (upright, leaning forward, hands on knees).
2. **Abnormal breath sounds**: Wheezes, rales (crackles), and/or rhonchi (snoring/whistling sounds).
3. **Abnormal depth of breathing**: Hypoventilation (too shallow) or hyperventilation (too deep).
4. **Abnormal rate of breathing**: Tachypnea (too fast) or bradypnea (too slow).
5. **Abnormal chest wall movement**: Splinting, asymmetric, paradoxical (chest wall/diaphragm move in during inhalation and out during exhalation—opposite of normal).
6. **Irregular breathing pattern**: May include periods of apnea (no breathing).

Patients with inadequate ventilation or apnea in which there is no breathing or only occasional gasping require ventilation assistance, such as with a pocket mask or bag-valve mask (BVM).

NEGATIVE-PRESSURE BREATHING VS. POSITIVE-PRESSURE BREATHING

Negative-pressure (normal) breathing:

- The movement downward of the diaphragm (triggered by the phrenic nerves) creates a negative pressure in the lungs, drawing air into them.
- Blood flows from the lungs to the heart and back and to the body at a steady rate in normal breathing.
- The epiglottis closes the esophagus during inhalation, preventing air from entering the stomach.

Positive-pressure breathing:

- Ventilation forces air into the lungs, and this can result in dysfunction of the diaphragm because it is responding to a change in pressure rather than stimulation by the phrenic nerve.
- Blood flow from the lungs is reduced, resulting in decreased cardiac (heart) output.
- The epiglottis may stay open during ventilation, allowing air into the stomach and increasing the risk of vomiting.

BAG-VALVE MASK (BVM)

Bag-valve mask (BVM) ventilation equipment used for positive-pressure ventilation (PPV) includes a mask, a ventilator bag, an oxygen reservoir bag, and an attachment for oxygen delivery. The correct mask size is important: The mask should not cover the chin. BVM is contraindicated if the airway is not patent, but it is used for abnormal breathing and for respiratory distress/failure. BVM requires two EMS personnel—one to control the mask and the other to control the bag. Steps are as follows:

1. Position oneself behind the patient's head, place the mask over the patient's nose and mouth, and make a tight seal by holding it in place with the thumbs and index fingers while the other fingers slide under the patient's jaw to lift the chin.
2. Squeeze the bag with inhalations initially for 5 to 10 breaths and then adjust the rate to at least 12 breaths per minute, slowly adjusting the rate and tidal volume delivered.

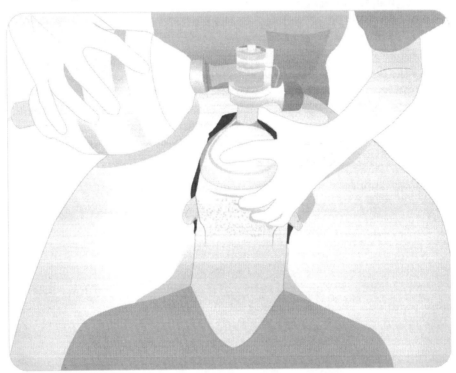

Assessment of lung compliance (the ability to expand and contract) includes observation of chest movement, rate of respirations, and the feel of BVM. Difficult ventilation suggests impaired compliance. Note: The BVM can be used with or without oxygen.

POCKET-MASK VENTILATION

Pocket-mask ventilation is used when administering cardiopulmonary resuscitation (CPR) to a patient who is in cardiac arrest and apneic (not breathing). If two EMS personnel are available, one should be positioned at the patient's head to administer pocket-mask ventilation while the other does compressions. If there is only one EMS personnel, then that person should be positioned at the patient's side. Administration is as follows:

1. Remove the mask from the container and push the flattened mask to open it.
2. Wipe the patient's face clean with alcohol swab if necessary to remove secretions, vomitus.
3. Do a chin tilt or jaw thrust and place the mask over the patient's nose and mouth, holding it in place with both hands to seal it tightly.

4. Take a deep breath and blow in through the one-way valve, watching the chest rise to ensure that ventilation has occurred.
5. Continue to ventilate the patient at a rate of 30 compressions to 2 ventilations for CPR.
6. Attach supplemental oxygen if available to improve oxygenation.
7. Upon patient recovery or completion of CPR, remove the mask, discard the valve, and disinfect the mask.

Pocket Mask

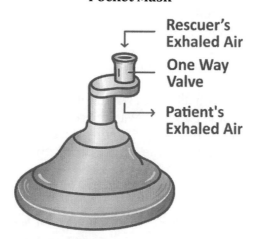

Rescuer's Exhaled Air

One Way Valve

Patient's Exhaled Air

Sellick's Maneuver (Cricoid Pressure)

Sellick's maneuver (cricoid pressure) may be used with PPV to prevent air from flowing down the esophagus and into the stomach rather than down the trachea and into the lungs because stomach distension increases the risk of vomiting. This maneuver may also be used with intubation to prevent regurgitation of stomach contents and aspiration. **Sellick's maneuver** may be used on unconscious patients receiving a mask or BVM. The procedure consists of applying pressure downward to the cricoid cartilage of the neck (which is at the bottom of the larynx and blocks the upper esophagus) with the thumb and index finger. Pressure is usually applied at 30 to 40 newtons but no greater than 40 newtons because too great of force may block the airway. The maneuver may also cause nausea and vomiting and, with severe pressure, may result in rupture of the esophagus. Vomiting is a contraindication.

Upper Airway Suctioning

Suctioning devices may be vehicle mounted or portable and should be checked to ensure that the tubing is intact and the canister has an airtight seal. Patients at risk for aspiration include those with an altered level of consciousness, those having difficulty swallowing or breathing, trauma patients, obese patients, and those with recurrent vomiting. **Oral suctioning** is used to remove secretions, vomitus, and blood. Suctioning may be done with a rigid-tip catheter (Yankauer) or a soft-tip catheter. Steps include the following:

1. Don a mask and gloves.
2. Measure the patient from the tip of the ear to the corner of the mouth to determine how far to insert the catheter.
3. Turn on the suction.
4. Use the cross-finger technique to open the mouth.
5. Insert the tube and apply suction. The rigid catheter has a finger control to start and stop suction.

6. Move the catheter around the gum line and over the tongue to the back of the mouth, but avoid stimulating the gag reflex.
7. Suction for no longer than 15 seconds at a time.

Note: Clear a small infant's airway by suctioning the nose with a bulb syringe.

PORTABLE OXYGEN CYLINDERS

Two commonly used sizes of **portable oxygen cylinders** are D tanks (M15; 350 L) and E tanks (M24; 625 L). The EMS provider should use protective equipment (goggles, gloves). The cylinder should be placed upright. A label over the holes on the top of the cylinder indicates that the cylinder is full. Remove the label, leaving the washers in place unless the washers are built into the regulator. Face the opening of the tank away and use the key to crack the cylinder by letting out a small amount of oxygen. Apply the regulator and slide it into place. Tighten and then open the cylinder to check for pressure (there should be at least 200 psi). Close the cylinder, attach the oxygen tubing to the regulator, set the oxygen flow to the correct number of liters, and then open the cylinder and administer oxygen to the patient. When discontinuing use of the cylinder, turn off the cylinder, remove the oxygen tubing, turn the oxygen flow setting up to bleed air from the regulator, and remove the regulator.

OXYGEN DELIVERY DEVICES

Oxygen delivery devices provide oxygen-enriched air. Ambient air is about 21% oxygen, so the fraction of inspired air (FiO_2) is 21%.

- **Nasal cannula (prongs)**: FiO_2 of 24–40% with flows of ≤6 liters per minute (LPM). Humidification should be used for prolonged flow rates of >4 LPM.
- **Partial rebreather face mask**: This mask covers the nose and mouth, delivering FiO_2 of 30–60%, but the flow of oxygen should be maintained at 6–12 LPM to decrease the risk of rebreathing. Because of the higher flow rate, humidification should be used.
- **Venturi mask**: Oxygen entrainment masks come with different-sized color-coded nozzles to more accurately control FiO_2, with different sizes providing different FiO_2 levels, usually ranging from 24–50%, although an FiO_2 reading of >35% is not always reliable. The flow rate is 12–15 LPM. Humidifiers may be used.
- **Non-rebreather mask**: This mask covers the mouth and nose with a reservoir bag of oxygen. A one-way valve prevents the patient from rebreathing exhaled air. FiO_2 is about 60–80% or greater at a flow rate of 15 LPM.

RECOVERY POSITION

The recovery position is used for patients who are unconscious but breathing (such as those with a drug overdose or after a seizure) and have no life-threatening injuries. This position helps to maintain a patent airway and reduces the risk of aspiration from vomitus.

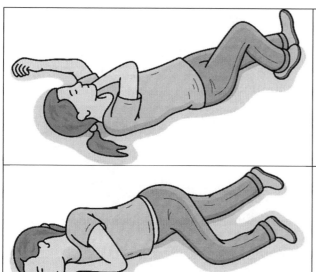	Kneeling beside the patient, lift his or her chin to ensure that the airway is open and place his or her closest arm at a right angle to the body with hand up. Place the patient's farthest arm around his or her neck with the hand touching the opposite cheek. Flex the patient's knee to 90° until the foot is flat on the floor/surface.
	Using the patient's knee as a fulcrum and supporting the farthest arm and shoulder, roll the patient onto his or her side by pulling on the farthest knee. Make sure that the top knee contacts the floor/surface to support the patient's body and that the top hand is under his or her head/neck to keep the neck in a neutral position.

ARTERIAL BLOOD GASES

Arterial blood gases are monitored to assess the effectiveness of oxygenation, ventilation, and acid-base status and to determine oxygen flow rates. The partial pressure of a gas is the pressure that is exerted by each gas in a mixture of gases, proportional to its concentration, based on total atmospheric pressure of 760 mmHg at sea level. Normal values include the following:

1. Acidity/alkalinity (pH): 7.35–7.45
2. Partial pressure of carbon dioxide ($PaCO_2$): 35–45 mmHg
3. Partial pressure of oxygen (PaO_2): 80 mmHg
4. Bicarbonate concentration (HCO_3): 22–26 mEq/L (a lower level is a base deficit, and a higher level is a base excess)
5. Oxygen saturation (SaO_2): ≥95%

The relationship between these elements, particularly the $PaCO_2$ and the PaO_2, indicates the respiratory status. For example, $PaCO_2$ >55 and PaO_2 <60 in a patient previously in good health indicates respiratory failure. There are many issues to consider. Ventilator management may require a higher $PaCO_2$ to prevent barotrauma and a lower PaO_2 to reduce oxygen toxicity.

ACID/BASE BALANCE

Respiratory acidosis: Hypoventilation (decreased breathing or inadequate mechanical ventilation) retains carbon dioxide and increases acid, which decreases the pH (acidity) to less than 7.35 (more acidic). The kidneys retain bicarbonate to compensate.

- **Causes**: COPD, pneumonia, muscle weakness, sedative/barbiturate overdose, obesity, muscle weakness (Guillain-Barré syndrome).
- **Symptoms**: Drowsiness, dizziness, headache, confusion, seizures, flushing, and low BP, tachypnea (tachy- = rapid; -pnea = breathing), tachycardia, and ventricular fibrillation.
- **Treatment**: Improved ventilation and bronchodilators.

Respiratory alkalosis: Hyperventilation (increased breathing) exhales more carbon dioxide and decreases acid, which increases the pH to greater than 7.45 (more alkalotic). The kidneys excrete increased bicarbonate to compensate.

- **Causes**: Hypoxia (low oxygen), brain injury, acetylsalicylic acid (ASA, i.e., aspirin) overdose, pulmonary embolism (clot), and septicemia.
- **Symptoms**: Confusion, lethargy, tachycardia, arrhythmia (irregular pulse), epigastric pain, nausea, and vomiting.
- **Treatment**: Identify and treat the underlying cause, and provide oxygen.

Metabolic acidosis: The kidneys excrete less acid, causing acid retention which decreases the pH, or the body excretes excess bicarbonate (through diarrhea), also decreasing the pH. Hyperventilation occurs in order to exhale additional carbon dioxide and acid to compensate.

- **Causes**: Diarrhea (it causes a loss of sodium bicarbonate), starvation, kidney disease, liver failure, excessive alcohol, shock, severe dehydration, and diabetic ketoacidosis (it causes acidic ketone bodies to build up).
- **Symptoms**: Headache, confusion, abnormal pulse, nausea, vomiting, diarrhea, and low BP.
- **Treatment**: Identify and treat the underlying cause. Bicarbonate is rarely administered, but it may be indicated in severe cases.

Metabolic alkalosis: Vomiting excretes excessive acid and/or the kidneys retain salt and potassium to compensate for vomiting, but in doing so, excrete more hydrogen ions (acid). This increases the body's pH, and hypoventilation occurs to retain carbon dioxide and acid.

- **Causes**: Excessive prolonged vomiting, low potassium level, advanced kidney failure.
- **Symptoms**: Confusion, anxiety, tremors, muscle cramping, seizures, tachycardia (rapid pulse), nausea, and vomiting.
- **Treatment**: Patient may respond to 0.9% IV saline (50-100 mL/hr.), but the underlying cause must be identified and treated. Some patients may require hemodialysis.

> **Review Video: Blood Gases**
> Visit mometrix.com/academy and enter code: 611909

OXYGEN VIA FACEMASK

Ensuring that a **facemask** (Ambu bag) is the correct fit and type is important for adequate ventilation, oxygenation, and prevention of aspiration. Difficulties in management of facemask ventilation relate to risk factors: >55 years, obesity, beard, edentulous, and history of snoring. In some cases, if dentures are adhered well, they may be left in place during induction. The facemask is applied by lifting the mandible (jaw thrust) to the mask and avoiding pressure on soft tissue. Oral or nasal airways may be used, ensuring that the distal end is at the angle of the mandible. There are a number of steps to prevent mask airway leaks:

- Increasing or decreasing the amount of air to the mask to allow better seal.
- Securing the mask with both hands while another person ventilates.
- Accommodating a large nose by using the mask upside down.
- Utilizing a laryngeal mask airway if excessive beard prevents seal.

VENTURI FACEMASK VENTILATION AND HUMIDIFIERS

The **Venturi facemask** is a high flow air-entrainment mask that mixes air and oxygen and provides a fixed flow of oxygen to the patient, usually ranging from FiO_2 of 24-50%, although FiO_2 above 35% is not always reliable. The mask comes with a set of different color-coded jets that control the mixture of air and oxygen in order to provide the desired oxygen concentration. The Venturi mask is used primarily with patients, such as those with COPD, who require oxygen supplementation but have a hypoxic drive to breathe and may be used if the EMS is concerned that the patient will retain carbon dioxide. The oxygen flow rate is set between 12 and 15 L/min.

The Venturi mask does not require the use of a **humidifier** because of the large amount of air mixed with the oxygen. However, a humidifier may be used if the patient has an artificial airway, such as a tracheostomy, as the humidification helps to loosen secretions, but the risk of infection increases. The oxygen flow rate must be between 10 and 15 L/min. Humidifiers are no longer routinely used with oxygen administration because studies show they have little effect on upper respiratory dryness.

NASOPHARYNGEAL AIRWAY (NPA)

The nasopharyngeal airway (NPA), a blind-insertion airway device, is indicated for unconscious or semiconscious patients who still have a gag reflex or those who cannot tolerate an oropharyngeal airway (OPA), but it should be avoided with severe head injury, risk of basal skull fracture, nasal bleeding, and history of deviated septum or nasal fracture. It's important to use the appropriate size. To insert the NPA, perform the following steps:

1. Choose a size that is slightly smaller in diameter than the patient's nostril.
2. Measure from the tip of the earlobe to the tip of the nose.
3. Lubricate the NPA with water-soluble lubricant and insert it in the larger and most patent (open) nostril. If inserting into the right nostril, insert with the bevel (tip) angled toward the nasal septum (the bony cartilage division between the nostrils). If inserting it into the left nostril, invert the NPA to angle the bevel toward the septum.
4. When the NPA reaches the throat, rotate it 180° into the proper position.

Nasopharyngeal Airway Placement

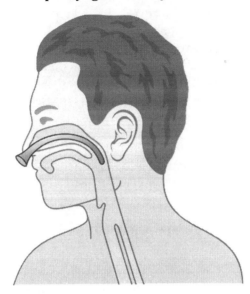

POSITIVE AIRWAY PRESSURE (PAP) DEVICES

All positive airway pressure (PAP) devices, such as **continuous positive airway pressure** (CPAP), have an air blower that delivers pressurized room air to an interface/mask. Pressure can be increased or decreased by adjusting the speed or the amount of airflow, with most machines generating from 2-20 cm of water pressure. Carbon dioxide is expelled through a vent or a nonrebreather valve on expiration. **Bilevel PAP (BiPAP, BPAP)** devices deliver two levels of pressure, which can be preset. Inspiratory PAP (IPAP) is set at a higher level (10 cmH$_2$O) than is expiratory PAP (EPAP) (5 cmH$_2$O) to allow a higher pressure needed to open the airway during inspiration but reduce the pressure to facilitate expiration. PAP is indicated for pulmonary edema, CHF, COPD, asthma, and near drowning.

The procedure includes the following:

1. Fill the humidifier with distilled water.
2. Program the settings.
3. Fit the mask and headgear/straps.
4. Begin with the pressure at the lowest setting, usually 5 cmH$_2$O (CPAP), and increase it slowly at 1 cmH$_2$O every few minutes until the optimal level is reached.
5. Monitor the oxygen saturation and respirations.

Respiratory Emergencies

ASSESSMENT OF LUNG SOUNDS

The lungs should be auscultated for normal and abnormal **breath sounds.**

- **Vesicular**: Normal low-pitched sound over lung bases and most lung fields.
- **Bronchovesicular**: Medium-pitched sound heard over the main bronchi. Duration is the same in expiration and inspiration.
- **Bronchial**: Normal high-pitched loud sound heard over the trachea. The expiratory sound is as long or longer than the inspiratory sound. It is abnormal if it is heard over the lung bases.
- **Rales (crackles)**: High-pitched crackles usually heard at the end of expiration in the lung bases, indicating fluid in the alveoli. May be fine or coarse.
- **Rhonchi**: Deep rumbling sound that may be high-pitched and sibilant (whistling) or low-pitched and sonorous (snoring) caused by constricted airways or large amounts of secretions in the airways. It is more pronounced on expiration.
- **Wheezes**: High- or low-pitched whistling or musical sounds most pronounced on expiration. They often indicate asthma or foreign-body obstruction.
- **Stridor**: Crowing sound caused by inflammation and swelling of the larynx and trachea. Common finding in croup (associated with cough).
- **Grunts**: Indicates respiratory distress in a newborn.
- **Friction rub**: Grating sound heard over the area of the lungs where the pleura is inflamed.

> **Review Video: Lung Sounds**
> Visit mometrix.com/academy and enter code: 765616

COMMON RESPIRATORY CONDITIONS

ASTHMA

Asthma is the result of an immune response that causes constriction of bronchi and inflammation and increased secretions in the lower airways. Symptoms include cough, wheezing, diminished breath sounds, dyspnea, and difficulty speaking. Children's symptoms are often intermittent, whereas adults' symptoms tend to be persistent. Death from asthma is most common in those older than 65. Geriatric patients are most at risk from influenza, pneumonia, and pneumococcal pneumonia.

Prehospital Interventions: Administer albuterol (nebulized/metered dose) per protocol and oxygen (6-8 L per minute), and provide airway management and ventilation. Provide CPAP for moderate/severe cases. If severe, provide rapid transport.

PERTUSSIS (WHOOPING COUGH)

Pertussis consists of a severe persistent whooping cough, thick sputum, post-cough emesis, petechiae on the upper body, and sclera from exertion. Infants may develop CNS damage, apnea, or pneumonia; children may develop hernia or muscle damage; and adults may develop hernia or a fractured rib.

Prehospital Interventions: Use standard and droplet precautions, provide the patient a position of comfort, and manage the patient's airway, ventilation, and oxygen supplementation as needed.

CYSTIC FIBROSIS (CF)

CF is a progressive congenital disease that particularly affects the pancreas and lungs, causing the production of thick mucus that clogs the lungs and causes recurrent bacterial infections of the lower respiratory tract. Symptoms include severe cough, sputum, fever, and dyspnea.

Prehospital Interventions: Use standard and droplet precautions, and provide the patient a position of comfort. Manage the patient's airway, ventilation, and oxygen supplementation. Start an IV access line. If severe, provide rapid transport.

CHRONIC PULMONARY OBSTRUCTIVE DISEASE (COPD)

COPD is a disease with limitations of airflow, narrowing airways, exertional dyspnea, chronic cough, right-sided heart failure (cor pulmonale), damaged and distended alveoli, barrel chest, and clubbed fingers. Symptoms include severe dyspnea, cough, sputum, cyanosis, and the tripod position. Specific types of COPD include:

- Chronic Bronchitis: Chronic inflammation of bronchial passages with cough and sputum production, resulting in narrowed airway passages and dyspnea. Symptoms usually persist for more than 3 months per year.
- Emphysema: Chronic inflammation of the alveoli of the lungs results in ruptures and large, distended air sacs that trap air. Symptoms include dyspnea, cyanosis, difficulty exhaling, barrel chest, altered mental status, and pursed-lip breathing.

Prehospital Interventions: Manage the patient's airway and ventilation and provide oxygen per nasal cannula or Venturi mask to maintain oxygen saturation >90%, provide the patient with a position of comfort or capnography near 35-45 mmHg, peak flow, and consider CPAP. Administer a beta-agonist bronchodilator (albuterol) according to protocol. Severe: Provide rapid transport.

PNEUMONIA

Pneumonia is inflammation of the lung, filling the alveoli with exudate and interfering with ventilation. It is common throughout childhood and adulthood. **Pneumonia** may be a primary disease, or it may occur secondary to another infection or disease, such as lung cancer. Pneumonia may be caused by bacteria, viruses, parasites, fungi, or toxins. Pneumonia is characterized by location (lobar, bronchial/lobular, interstitial). Symptoms include fever, chills, cough, purulent sputum, and difficulty breathing, chest pain on cough or deep inhalation, and headache. Bacterial pneumonia is treated with antibiotics, and viral pneumonia is treated with antivirals. Geriatric patients may exhibit confusion. Pediatric patients with undeveloped or poor immune systems, or chronic illnesses such as cystic fibrosis and asthma, have an increased risk.

Prehospital Interventions: Use standard and droplet precautions, including wearing a protective face mask. Place the patient in a position of comfort (usually with his or her head elevated), manage the airway and ventilation, provide supplemental oxygen, and provide IV access line if indicated.

> **Review Video: Pneumonia**
> Visit mometrix.com/academy and enter code: 628264

Spontaneous Pneumothorax

Spontaneous pneumothorax is air in the pleural space that causes the lung to collapse but without an obvious cause. Symptoms include an abrupt onset of sharp chest pain on the affected side, dyspnea, difficulty breathing, and decreased or absent respirations on the affected side.

- **Primary** (no underlying lung disease): It is most common in tall, thin adolescents and young adults and is associated with cigarette smoking. It often resolves without treatment and rarely progresses to tension pneumothorax.
- **Secondary** (underlying lung disease): It is most common in those with chronic obstructive pulmonary disease (COPD), cystic fibrosis, and severe asthma, and it poses a risk of death because of respiratory compromise. Patients may develop hypoxemia, altered mental status, coma, and tension pneumothorax.

Prehospital Interventions: Manage the patient's airway, ventilation, and oxygen supplementation. Place the patient in a position of comfort and transport. A large spontaneous pneumothorax will require catheter aspiration of air or insertion of a chest tube.

Pulmonary Edema

Pulmonary edema occurs when the alveoli in the lungs fill with fluid.

- **Cardiogenic**: The left ventricle weakens, so the heart cannot pump adequate amounts of blood, resulting in back pressure in the left atrium and the vessels in the lungs, forcing fluid into the alveoli. Left ventricular damage can result from coronary artery disease, cardiomyopathy, myocardial infarction, defective heart valves, and uncontrolled hypertension.
- **Non-cardiogenic**: Damage to the capillaries in the lungs causes them to leak fluid into the alveoli. Conditions causing noncardiogenic pulmonary edema include acute respiratory distress syndrome (ARDS), adverse drug reactions, pulmonary embolism, lung injury, viral infections, nervous system conditions, toxin exposure, smoke inhalation, near drowning, and high-altitude pulmonary edema (HAPE).

Symptoms include severe dyspnea, orthopnea, tachycardia, cough, and chest pain.

Prehospital Interventions: Manage airway, ventilation, and supplemental oxygen/CPAP or intubation with PEEP, and start an IV access line. Medications may include dopamine, dobutamine, nitroglycerin, and furosemide (per protocol). Severe cases require rapid transport. For HAPE, immediately descend to a lower altitude (500-1000 m), provide supplemental oxygen and a portable hyperbaric chamber, and administer acetazolamide or dexamethasone (per protocol).

Epiglottitis

Acute epiglottitis (supraglottitis) occurs in children (primarily 1-8 years old) and in young adults. Acute epiglottitis requires immediate medical attention because it can rapidly become obstructive. The onset is usually very sudden and often occurs during the night. The patient may awaken suddenly with a fever, but he or she usually does not have a cough.

Symptoms include the following:

- **Tripod position**: Sits upright, leaning forward with the chin out, mouth open, and tongue protruding.
- **Agitation**: Appears restless, tense, and agitated.
- **Drooling**: Excess secretions combined with pain or dysphagia and a mouth-open position cause drooling.
- **Voice**: No hoarseness, but the voice sounds thick and "froglike."
- **Cyanosis**: Color is usually pale and sallow initially but may progress to frank cyanosis.
- **Throat**: On examination, the epiglottis appears bright red and swollen. Note: The patient's throat should not be examined with a tongue blade unless intubation and tracheostomy equipment are immediately available because the examination can trigger an obstruction.

Prehospital Interventions: Provide rapid transport, administer high-flow oxygen with a blow-by mask, or provide slow ventilation with a BVM.

ACUTE PULMONARY EMBOLISM

Acute pulmonary embolism occurs when a pulmonary artery or arteriole is blocked by a blood clot originating in the venous system or the right heart. While most **pulmonary emboli** are from thrombus formation, other causes may be air, fat, or septic embolus. Common originating sites for thrombus formation are the deep veins in the legs, the pelvic veins, and the right atrium. Causes include atrial fibrillation and stasis related to damage to the endothelial wall and changes in blood coagulation factors. Symptoms include dyspnea, tachypnea, tachycardia, anxiety, restlessness, chest pain, fever, rales, cough (sometimes with hemoptysis), and hemodynamic instability.

Prehospital Interventions: Assess vital signs, oxygen saturation, lung sounds, signs of jugular vein distention, signs of DVT, and signs of shock. Provide the patient with high-flow oxygen per nasal cannula (C-PAP or BIPAP if hypoxia persists), insert a large bore IV line in the antecubital fossa (to facilitate CT scan with dye), administer NS if the patient is hypotensive but limit to 500-1000 mL to avoid pulmonary edema. Monitor ECG, typical pattern is S1Q3T3—elevated S wave (lead 1) and Q wave and inverted T wave (lead III). Provide analgesia per protocol (avoid morphine). Administer norepinephrine for persistent hypotension. Provide immediate anticoagulation, such as IV heparin, if available.

Cardiology and Resuscitation

Cardiovascular Emergencies

CIRCULATORY SYSTEM

The circulatory system controls blood flow throughout the body and to the tissues, controls gas exchange (carbon dioxide and oxygen), serves as a reservoir for blood, maintains blood pH through a buffer system, responds to infections, and facilitates coagulation (blood clotting). The circulatory system includes the cardiovascular system (heart and blood vessels) and the blood.

- **Heart**: The heart has four chambers, upper (right atrium and left atrium) and lower (right ventricle and left ventricle). The heart muscle receives blood from two major coronary arteries and their branches. The myocardium (heart muscle) receives blood from two major coronary arteries and their branches. The inner lining of the heart is the endocardium, and the lining that surrounds the heart is the pericardium, which has an inner double-layered serous membrane (visceral pericardium) and a fibrous outer layer (parietal pericardium).
- **Vessels**: The venous system includes veins, venules, and venous capillaries and brings blood back to the heart via the inferior and superior vena cava. The arterial system, including the coronary arteries, branches from the aorta after it leaves the heart and includes arteries, arterioles, and arterial capillaries.
- **Blood**: Blood consists of red blood cells (erythrocytes); white blood cells (leukocytes including monocytes, lymphocytes, basophils, neutrophils, and eosinophils); platelets (thrombocytes); and plasma, the liquid portion of the blood (which contains clotting factors).

> **Review Video: Functions of the Circulatory System**
> Visit mometrix.com/academy and enter code: 376581

CONDUCTION SYSTEM OF THE HEART

Normal conduction of the heart has the following four stages:

1. **Generation of an impulse at the sinoatrial (SA) node** (primary pacemaker) located at the junction of the right atrium and superior vena cava: The electrical impulse travels the cells of the atria along internodal pathways, causing electrical stimulation and contraction of the atria, including Bachmann's bundle, which stimulates the left atrium.
2. **Atrioventricular node conduction of impulse**: This occurs when the impulses from the SA node reach the AV node in the right atrial wall near the tricuspid valve. There is a slight delay (about one-tenth of a second), allowing the atria to empty.
3. **Atrioventricular bundle (bundle of His) conduction**: The AV node relays the impulse to the ventricles through the atrioventricular bundle—specialized conduction cells in the ventricular septum that branch to the right and left ventricles, carrying the electrical impulse.
4. **Purkinje fiber conduction**: Impulses are conducted down the AV bundles to the base of the heart where they divide into the Purkinje fibers, which stimulate the myocardial cells to contract the ventricles.

CARDIAC CYCLE AND BLOOD FLOW THROUGH THE HEART

The cardiac cycle involves one complete heartbeat with systole (ventricular contraction) and diastole (relaxation) phases. **Stroke volume** is the volume of blood ejected from the left ventricle in one cardiac cycle (about 60–70 mL), and **cardiac output** is the heart rate times the stroke volume.

The **blood flows** as follows:

- Deoxygenated venous blood returns to the heart per the inferior vena cava, superior vena cava, and coronary sinus (bringing blood from the coronary arteries) into the right atrium, and then it flows through the tricuspid valve into the right ventricle.
- From the right ventricle, blood flows through the pulmonic (semilunar) valve into the pulmonary artery and to the lungs to exchange carbon dioxide for oxygen.
- Oxygenated blood flows from the lungs through the pulmonary veins into the left atrium and through the mitral (bicuspid) valve into the left ventricle.
- From the left ventricle, blood flows through the aortic valve and into the aorta, the coronary arteries, and the general circulation through the thoracic and abdominal aorta.
- After blood flows through the valves, they close to prevent backflow. Both atria and both ventricles contract simultaneously.

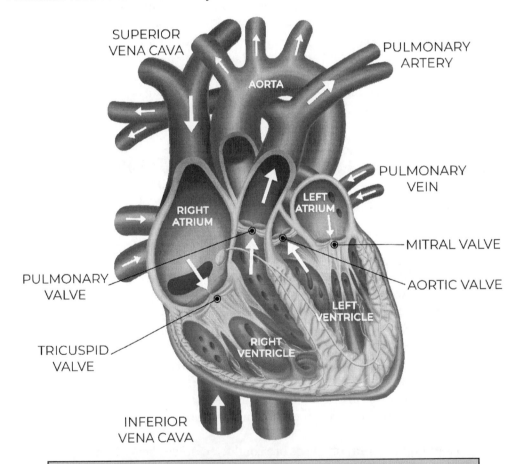

Review Video: <u>Heart Blood Flow</u>
Visit mometrix.com/academy and enter code: 783139
Review Video: <u>Diastolic vs Systolic</u>
Visit mometrix.com/academy and enter code: 898934

PERFUSION, OXYGENATION OF TISSUES, AND CARDIAC COMPROMISE

Perfusion depends on an adequate supply of red blood cells, which carry oxygen. Perfusion may be impaired if the heart does not pump adequately, if the rate of heart contractions is too low or too rapid to be effective, and if the volume of blood and/or red blood cells pumped is not adequate to provide oxygenation to the tissues. With adequate perfusion, **oxygenation of tissues** occurs when blood flows throughout the body, and gas exchange of carbon dioxide and waste products for oxygen occurs at the capillaries. **Cardiac compromise** results in inadequate circulation and/or perfusion of vital organs. Cardiac compromise may result from atherosclerosis (plaques/fatty deposits) in the arterial lumens, resulting in obstructed blood flow and inadequate dilation and constriction of arteries. Ischemia (low oxygenation) occurs with decreased blood flow and can damage tissues, but occlusion (obstruction) can result in the death of tissue. Cardiac compromise may result from heart damage causing an inadequate heart rate and/or pumping. Cardiac compromise may also result from an inadequate volume of circulating blood.

OBTAINING A MANUAL BLOOD PRESSURE

When obtaining **a** manual blood pressure, a correctly sized cuff is essential. The cuff width should be 40% of the circumference (or 20% wider than the diameter) of the middle of the limb to which the blood pressure cuff will be applied. The bladder (which fills with air as the cuff is inflated) should circle at least 80% of the limb and the cuff width (when used on the upper arm) should cover two-thirds of the length of the upper arm. Small or extra-large blood pressure cuffs may be indicated. Cuffs should not be applied to a limb receiving IV fluids or one that is traumatized. The forearm (or leg) should be at heart level and the hand turned up if using an arm. Procedure:

1. Palpate brachial or peripheral artery, deflate cuff completely, and apply snugly to the site (two fingers should be able to fit between the cuff and arm), aligning the centering arrows correctly or centering the bladder over the artery. Cuff should be one-inch above site of arterial pulsation (popliteal or antecubital).
2. Inflate bladder and increase pressure to about 30 mmHg above anticipated base or 30 mmHg above where pulse is no longer palpable.
3. Slowly release air and note when heart sound appears (systolic) and when it disappears (diastolic).
4. Record BP reading.

ANGINA

Chest pain may indicate **angina** (pain from temporary constriction/blockage of blood flow in the coronary arteries) or a heart attack (pain caused by blockage of blood flow to the heart muscle because of a blood clot (most common) or hemorrhage, resulting in the death of heart tissue). Heart problems in children are often associated with congenital heart disease. Geriatric and female patients may not have chest pain with a heart attack. Make note of the following:

- Character, location, and severity of the pain.
- Radiation of pain to the neck, jaw, arms, back, jaw, and/or stomach.
- Shortness of breath at rest, with exertion, or worsening when lying flat.
- Cold, clammy skin is common with a heart attack.
- Note BP, pulse (rapid, irregular, slow), and respirations.
- Note nausea and/or vomiting and dizziness/lightheadedness.

ANGINA PECTORIS (STABLE)

Impairment of blood flow through the coronary arteries leads to ischemia of the cardiac muscle and **angina pectoris**—pain that may occur in the sternum, chest, neck, arms (especially the left arm), or back. The pain frequently occurs with crushing pain substernally, radiating down the left arm or both arms, although this type of pain is more common in males than females, whose symptoms may appear less acute and may include nausea, shortness of breath, and fatigue. Elderly or diabetic patients may also have pain in their arms, no pain at all (silent ischemia), or weakness and numbness in both arms.

Stable angina episodes usually last for <5 minutes and are fairly predictable, exercise-induced episodes caused by atherosclerotic lesions blocking >75% of the lumen of the affected coronary artery. Precipitating events include exercise, a decrease in the environmental temperature, heavy eating, strong emotions (such as fright or anger), or exertion, including coitus. Stable angina episodes usually resolve in less than 5 minutes by decreasing the activity level and administering sublingual nitroglycerin. Provide supportive care, oxygen, and assist the patient to take nitroglycerin if available.

ANGINA PECTORIS (UNSTABLE, VARIANT/PRINZMETAL'S)

Unstable angina (also known as preinfarction or crescendo angina) is a progression of coronary artery disease, and it occurs when there is a change in the pattern of stable angina. The pain may increase, may not respond to a single nitroglycerin dose, and may persist for >5 minutes. Usually pain is more frequent, lasts longer, and may occur at rest when sitting or lying down. Unstable angina may indicate a rupture of an atherosclerotic plaque and the beginning of thrombus formation, so it should always be treated as a medical emergency with rapid transport because it may indicate a myocardial infarction.

Variant angina (also known as **Prinzmetal's angina**) results from spasms of the coronary arteries. It can be associated with or without atherosclerotic plaques and is often related to smoking, alcohol, or illicit stimulants. Variant angina frequently occurs cyclically at the same time each day and often while the person is at rest. Nitroglycerin or calcium channel blockers are used for treatment.

MANAGEMENT OF A PATIENT WITH ANGINA

Management of a patient with angina begins with a thorough assessment, primary and secondary survey, and use of the OPQRST and SAMPLE methods of history taking. Patients are often very frightened, so the EMS provider should provide clear feedback and reassurance. The patient should be placed in the semi-Fowler's position, especially if he or she is experiencing shortness of breath, and the oxygen saturation should be monitored. Respiratory compromise may require supplemental oxygen, bag-mask ventilation (BVM) assistance, PEEP, CPAP/BiPAP, manually triggered ventilators (MTVs), or automatic transport ventilators (ATVs). If an EMT is the first to arrive at the scene, the EMT should determine the need for the assistance of an advanced emergency medical technician (AEMT) or a paramedic.

Pharmacological interventions (assist the patient with medication administration, or administer the medication according to protocol) may include the following:

- **Aspirin** (for suspected heart attack; Bayer, Heartline, ZORprin, Empirin): Provide 162 to 325 mg chewable (preferred). Contraindicated with GI bleeding, stroke.
- **Nitroglycerin** (for suspected angina; Nitro-Dur, Nitrolingual, NitroMist): Provide 0.4 mg sublingually repeated every 3–5 minutes up to three doses. Contraindicated if the patient has recently taken Viagra, had a stroke, or has excessive bleeding.
- **Oral glucose** (for suspected hypoglycemia/insulin reaction): Glucose tablets, solution.

All patients with chest pain should be transported because even mild chest discomfort may indicate that the patient is having a heart attack, especially in older patients and female patients, who often have atypical symptoms.

MYOCARDIAL INFARCTION

Myocardial infarction (also referred to as an MI or heart attack) may occur after an episode of unstable angina caused by a rupture of an atherosclerotic plaque and thrombosis associated with coronary artery spasm, but it may also result from vasoconstriction, acute blood loss, decreased oxygen, and ingestion of cocaine. Symptoms may vary considerably, with males having the more "classic" symptom of a sudden onset of crushing chest pain. Elderly and diabetic patients may complain primarily of weakness. Symptoms include the following:

- Angina with pain in the chest that may radiate to the neck or arms, crushing pain, tightness (often more than 30 minutes and unrelieved by rest or nitroglycerin).
- Hypertension or hypotension.
- Palpitations, tachycardia, bradycardia, and dysrhythmias.
- Dyspnea.
- ECG changes (ST segment and T-wave changes), tachycardia, bradycardia, and dysrhythmias.
- Pulmonary edema, peripheral edema, weak/absent peripheral pulses.
- Nausea and vomiting.
- Pallor, cold and clammy skin, diaphoresis.
- Neurological/psychological disturbances: Anxiety, light-headedness, headache, visual abnormalities, slurred speech, and fear.

Prehospital Interventions: Manage the patient's airway/ventilation/oxygen supplementation, provide supportive care, perform CPR/defibrillation if needed, and provide rapid transport.

> **Review Video: Myocardial Infarction**
> Visit mometrix.com/academy and enter code: 148923

ECG ANALYSIS OF MYOCARDIAL INFARCTION

Myocardial ischemia results in ST-segment depression and T-wave inversion. **Myocardial injury** results in ST-segment elevation and T-wave inversion. **Myocardial infarction** results in hyperacute T waves (initial stage), ST-segment elevation, T-wave inversion, and pathologic Q waves. Arrhythmias common to MI include sinus tachycardia (rapid heart rate), sinus bradycardia (slow heart rate), heart blocks, ventricular fibrillation, pulseless electrical activity (PEA), and asystole. Rapid transport is indicated for patients having no relief from medication, hypotension, hypoperfusion, and/or significant ECG changes/abnormalities. No transport is indicated only for patient refusal.

Q wave MI:

- Characterized by a series of abnormal Q waves (wider and deeper) on ECG, especially in the early morning (related to adrenergic activity)
- Infarction is usually prolonged and results in necrosis (This may indicate extensive transient ischemia)
- Usually transmural

Non-Q wave MI:

- Characterized by changes in the ST-T wave with ST depression (usually reversible within a few days)
- Usually reperfusion occurs spontaneously, so the infarct size is smaller; contraction necrosis related to reperfusion is common
- Usually nontransmural

ELECTROCARDIOGRAM (ECG)

The electrocardiogram (ECG) records and shows a graphic display of the electrical activity of the heart through a number of different waveforms, complexes, and intervals as follows:

- **P wave**: Start of the electrical impulse in the sinus node and spreading through the atria, muscle depolarization
- **QRS complex**: Ventricular muscle depolarization and atrial repolarization
- **T wave**: Ventricular muscle repolarization (resting state) as cells regain a negative charge
- **U wave**: Repolarization of the Purkinje fibers

A modified lead II ECG is often used to monitor basic heart rhythms and dysrhythmias. Typical placement of leads for a two-lead ECG is 3 to 5 cm inferior to the right clavicle and left lower rib cage. Typical placement for a three-lead ECG is the right arm (RA) near the shoulder, the V_5 position over the fifth intercostal space (LA), and the left upper leg (LL) near the groin.

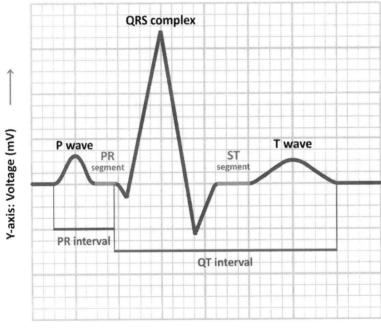

12-LEAD ELECTROCARDIOGRAPHY

The most common electrocardiography setup is the **12-lead ECG**, which assesses 12 different views of the heart. The 12-lead ECG actually comprises 10 electrodes and 12 sources of measurement as follows:

- Four limb electrodes: right and left arm and right and left leg (RA, LA, RL, LL). Put in place, avoiding heavily muscled areas.
- Six precordial (in front of the heart/pericardium) electrodes:
  - V1—Right sternum, fourth intercostal space
  - V2—Left sternum, fourth intercostal space
  - V3—Halfway between V2 and V4
  - V4—Midclavicular line, fifth intercostal space
  - V5—In line with V4 at the anterior axillary line
  - V6—In line with V4 and V5 at the midaxillary line

The patient should be placed in the flat supine position for the ECG, although he or she can sit in the semi-Fowler's position if unable to tolerate a flat position. The skin should be dry and the hair clipped or shaved to improve the electrode contact, and conductive gel is applied to the electrode. The skin can be wiped with an alcohol pad to remove oils or other residue before applying the electrodes. Electrodes should not be placed directly over a bone.

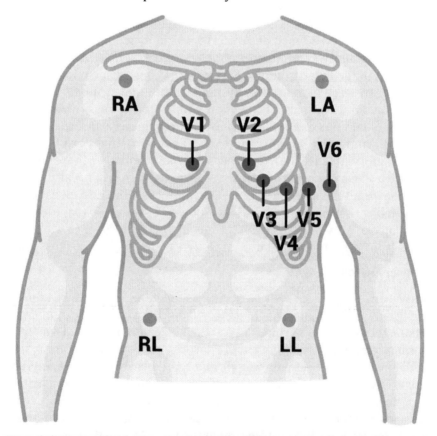

Review Video: Cardiovascular Assessment
Visit mometrix.com/academy and enter code: 323076

47

HEART SOUNDS

Normal and abnormal heart sounds include the following:

- **First and second sounds**: The first heart sound (S1—"lub") is closure of the mitral and tricuspid valves (heard at the apex/left ventricular area of the heart). The second heart sound (S2—"dub") is closure of the aortic and pulmonic valves (heard at the base of the heart). There may be a slight splitting of the S2.
- **Gallop rhythms**:
  - S3 occurs after S2 in children and young adults, but it may indicate heart failure or left ventricular failure in older adults (heard with the patient lying on the left side).
  - S4 occurs before S1 and occurs with ventricular hypertrophy, such as from coronary artery disease, hypertension, or aortic valve stenosis.
- **Opening snap**: Unusual, high-pitched sound occurring after S2 with stenosis of mitral valve from rheumatic heart disease
- **Ejection click**: Brief, high-pitched sound occurring immediately after S1 with stenosis of the aortic valve
- **Friction rub**: Harsh, grating sound heard in systole and diastole with pericarditis
- **Murmur**: Sound caused by turbulent blood flow from stenotic or malfunctioning valves, congenital defects, or increased blood flow

HEART FAILURE

Heart failure (HF, aka congestive HF) includes disorders of contractions (systolic "left-sided" dysfunction) or filling (diastolic dysfunction) or both, which result in hypertrophy (thickening, enlarging, and stiffening) of the myocardium (heart muscle). The most common causes are coronary artery disease, myocardial infarction, systemic or pulmonary hypertension, cardiomyopathy, and valvular disorders. The incidence of HF correlates with age. Left-sided HF may cause pulmonary edema that impairs ventilation, leading to hypoxia, especially when the patient is lying in a supine position, and right-sided HF may cause abdominal and peripheral edema of the feet and legs. The circulatory time with HF decreases overall, so changes in oximetry to show hypoxia may be delayed. The autonomic nervous system's regulation of breathing to control oxygen levels may be impaired, resulting in periodic breathing patterns, Cheyne-Stokes breathing, or central sleep apnea. Medications used to treat HF include ACE inhibitors (captopril, lisinopril), angiotensin receptor blockers (ARBs) (losartan, valsartan), beta-blockers (metoprolol, carvedilol), aldosterone agonists (spironolactone), and diuretics (hydrochlorothiazide, furosemide).

CHRONIC VS ACUTE HEART FAILURE

Chronic heart failure develops insidiously over time as the heart muscles weaken and enlarge, so initially patients may only note fatigue, weight gain, and swelling in their feet and ankles. **Acute heart failure** is characterized by impairment of gas exchange and decreased cardiac output because of changes in preload, contractibility, and heart rhythm; symptoms are more acute and may include irregular heartbeat, chest pain, cough, and rapid breathing, wheezing, and cyanosis from lack of adequate oxygen. Patients may also suffer from anxiety, decreased activity tolerance, and disturbances in sleep patterns. Medical management is aimed at increasing cardiac function, providing support, and monitoring treatment. Patients often are acutely short of breath and sitting upright, with rales evident in their lungs. Assessment includes conducting primary and secondary surveys, taking a complete medical history including medication use and home oxygen use, and assessing the patient's level of consciousness, airway status (cough, sputum, labored breathing, tripod position), heart rate/rhythm, peripheral pulses, edema (pitting/nonpitting, ascites, sacral), and complications.

48

Prehospital Interventions: Manage the patient's airway/ventilation/oxygen supplementation with a nonrebreather mask or BVM with high-flow oxygen. Position the mask for comfort and suction if necessary.

HYPERTENSIVE CRISIS

Hypertensive crisis (aka malignant hypertension) is a marked elevation in BP that can cause severe organ damage if left untreated. Causes include encephalopathy, intracranial hemorrhage, aortic dissection, eclampsia, and heart failure. Classifications are as follows:

- **Hypertensive emergency**: Acute hypertension, usually >120 mmHg diastolic, must be treated immediately to lower the BP in order to prevent damage to vital organs, such as the heart, brain, or kidneys.
- **Hypertensive urgency**: Acute hypertension must be treated within a few hours, but the vital organs are not in immediate danger. The blood pressure is lowered more slowly to avoid hypotension, ischemia of vital organs, or failure of autoregulation with a one-third reduction in 6 hours.

Symptoms include headache, dizziness, dyspnea, weakness, visual disturbances, anxiety, chest pain (atypical), heart failure, acute coronary syndrome, and stroke.

Prehospital Interventions: Asymptomatic hypertension requires referral to a physician, whereas severe symptoms require rapid transport. Interventions include airway support/ventilation with oxygen supplementation and advanced life support as needed. Patients with severe dyspnea and pulmonary edema may need CPAP.

THROMBOEMBOLISM AND PULMONARY EMBOLISM

Thromboembolism includes the formation of a thrombus (such as in the heart with atrial fibrillation and in the deep veins with immobilization) and an embolism in which a clot breaks off and travels through the circulatory system. Although thromboembolism may cause a heart attack or stroke, the most common presentation is a **pulmonary embolism (PE)** resulting from deep vein thrombosis. The patient may or may not complain of pain at the thrombus site, which may be swollen and erythematous (red), typically in a lower extremity. When the patient develops PE, the usual presentation is acute onset of dyspnea and tachycardia and sitting in the tripod position. Some patients may have ECG abnormalities, frothy sputum, cough, fever, hemoptysis, and jugular vein distension.

Prehospital Interventions: Provide supportive care, manage the patient's airway/ventilation/intubation as needed with oxygen to maintain oxygen saturation >94%, establish an IV access line, administer up to 1 L of NS, and give norepinephrine if indicated. If protocol permits, administer heparin for PE.

Shock and Resuscitation

SYMPTOMS AND INTERVENTIONS FOR SHOCK

Shock is a life-threatening condition that occurs when the tissues do not receive adequate oxygen, such as with severe bleeding or fluid loss, severe infection, heart failure, or abnormal dilation of the blood vessels. Indications of shock include extreme thirst; anxiety and restlessness; weak, rapid pulse; altered mental status progressing to loss of consciousness; rapid, shallow respirations; hypotension (low BP—often a late sign); and cool, clammy, pale skin with mottling sometimes on the extremities from inadequate perfusion. If left untreated, shock may lead to cardiac arrest. Note that geriatric patients may have a higher baseline respiration and heart rate and an irregular pulse.

Prehospital Interventions: Apply pressure to control the bleeding, perform spinal stabilization if needed, place the patient in the shock position (flat with feet elevated above the level of the heart, 8-12 inches), manage the patient's airway and ventilation and administer high-concentration oxygen, provide warming blankets to maintain the body temperature, provide reassurance, apply a pneumatic anti-shock garment (PASG), insert an IV access line, and administer fluids for hemorrhage/severe hypotension. Provide rapid transport if needed.

STAGES AND TYPES OF SHOCK

Shock generally occurs in stages as the body tries to compensate. **Compensated shock** occurs in the early stage while the body speeds up the heart rate and respirations and diverts blood to the vital organs (resulting in pale, cool skin) to maintain adequate perfusion and BP. **Decompensated shock** occurs when the body can no longer compensate and the BP falls and symptoms worsen. With irreversible shock, recovery is no longer possible because of cell damage caused by inadequate oxygenation and perfusion. **Types of shock** include the following:

- **Cardiogenic**: Heart failure, myocardial infarction, drug overdose, dysrhythmia, congenital heart disease
- **Distributive**: Anaphylaxis, drug overdose
- **Hypovolemic**: Hemorrhage, severe vomiting and/or diarrhea, severe burns, dehydration
- **Obstructive**: Pneumothorax, pericardial tamponade
- **Neurogenic**: Spinal cord injury (a form of distributive shock because of decreased vascular tone)
- **Septic**: Sepsis, severe infections (also a form of distributive shock)

Signs and symptoms are similar for all types of shock even though the mechanisms are different (excluding neurogenic shock which can present with bradycardia instead of tachycardia).

HYPOVOLEMIC SHOCK

Hypovolemic shock occurs when the total circulating volume of fluid decreases, leading to a fall in venous return that in turn causes a decrease in ventricular filling and preload. This results in a decrease in stroke volume and cardiac output. This in turn causes generalized arterial vasoconstriction, increasing afterload (increased systemic vascular resistance), and causing decreased tissue perfusion.

Hypovolemic shock is **classified** according to the degree of fluid loss as follows:

- **Class I**: <750 mL or ≤15% of total circulating volume (TCV) (usually well tolerated)
- **Class II**: 750-1500 mL or 15-30% of TCV (tachycardia, anxiety, narrow pulse pressure, and increased respirations)
- **Class III**: 1500-2000 mL or 30-40% of TCV (hypotension, pallor, cold, clammy skin, delayed capillary refill, severe tachycardia, and altered mental status)
- **Class IV**: >2000 mL or >40% of TCV (severe shock, a weak thready pulse, cyanosis, and death without aggressive resuscitation)

Prehospital Interventions: Control the patient's bleeding upon arrival to the scene. The EMS provider should insert two large-bore, short IV catheters, give 250-500 cc of warm isotonic boluses (20-30 mL/kg), keep the patient warm, maintain the patient's airway/ventilation/oxygen supplementation to maintain oxygen saturation at 90-92%, maintain the systolic BP at 70-90 mmHg, place him or her in the shock position, and provide rapid transport.

RESPIRATORY FAILURE/ARREST

Respiratory failure occurs when ventilation is insufficient for adequate gas exchange so that levels of carbon dioxide in the blood increase and levels of oxygen decrease. **Respiratory failure** may result from respiratory infection (pneumonia, tuberculosis), heart failure, chronic respiratory illness (asthma, chronic bronchitis, COPD), trauma, and depression of the CNS (usually from medications or trauma). Respiratory failure may be acute with sudden onset or chronic, developing over time. If untreated, respiratory failure can lead to **respiratory arrest**, which in turn leads to cardiac arrest. Indications of respiratory failure include altered mental status, cyanosis, labored breathing (dyspnea and orthopnea), coughing, fatigue, diminished breath sounds, and the presence of rales (crackles) and rhonchi (snoring/whistling sound). Patients may have hemoptysis (bloody sputum). The patient's oxygen saturation level is lower than 90% per pulse oximeter.

Prehospital Interventions: Manage the patient's airway/ventilation/oxygen supplementation; positive-pressure ventilation may be needed. Place the patient in a position of comfort (usually high Fowler's).

HEIMLICH MANEUVER FOR CHOKING
INFANTS

Indications of choking in **infants younger than 1 year old** include lack of breathing, gasping, cyanosis, and the inability to cry. The procedure for **Heimlich chest thrusts** includes the following:

- Position the infant in the prone position along your forearm with the infant's head lower than the trunk, being sure to support the head so the airway is not blocked.
- Using the heel of the hand, deliver five forceful upward blows between the shoulder blades.
- Sandwich the child between your two arms, and turn the infant into the supine position and drape over your thigh with his or her head lower than the trunk and the head supported.
- Using two fingers (as for CPR compressions), give up to five thrusts (about 1.5 inches deep) to the lower third of the sternum.
- Only do a finger sweep and remove a foreign object if the object is visible. Repeat five back blows, five chest thrusts until the foreign body is ejected.
- If the infant loses consciousness, begin CPR. If a pulse is noted but spontaneous respirations are absent, continue with ventilation only.

CHILDREN AND ADULTS

The universal sign of choking is when a person clutches his or her throat and appears to be choking or gasping for breath. If the person can speak ("Can you speak?") or cough, the Heimlich maneuver is not usually necessary. The Heimlich maneuver can be done with the victim sitting, standing, or supine. The Heimlich maneuver for **children (≥1 year) and adults** is as follows:

- Wrap both arms around the victim's waist from the back if sitting or standing. Make a fist and place the thumb side against the victim's abdomen slightly above the umbilicus. Grasp this hand with the other and thrust sharply upward to force air out of the lungs.
- Repeat as needed.
- If the victim loses consciousness, ease him or her into a supine position on the floor, and initiate chest compressions (CPR). Assess the airway and remove any visible obstruction. The blind finger sweep is no longer recommended. Repeat compressions and ventilations until recovery or emergency personnel arrive.

CARDIOPULMONARY RESUSCITATION (CPR) FOR CARDIAC ARREST

Cardiac arrest of unknown cause in adults or children is usually treated as though it were ventricular fibrillation or pulseless ventricular tachycardia, but the protocol varies. **Cardiopulmonary resuscitation (CPR)** involves the following components:

- Immediate defibrillation is performed according to protocol with an AED/manual defibrillator (preferred) followed by CPR, beginning with compressions (30:2 compression to ventilation at the rate of 100-120 per minute at least 2 inches deep; two-finger compressions, to one-third of the chest depth for infants and children) for 2 minutes or 5 cycles and repeat defibrillation.
- Repeat cycles of 2 minutes of CPR and defibrillation. (Laypeople may use compression-only CPR.)
- If a defibrillator is not readily available, CPR may begin first. Note that if a BVM is used, the break in compressions should not exceed 10 seconds. If an advanced airway/intubation is in place, ventilation should be at the rate of 8-10 per minute, maintaining oxygen saturation ≥94% but <100% with ventilation between compressions.
- The $ETCO_2$ value should be 10-20 mmHg if chest compressions are adequate, increasing to 35-45 mmHg with the return of spontaneous circulation (ROSC).

DEFIBRILLATION USING AN AUTOMATED/SEMI-AUTOMATED DEFIBRILLATOR

Emergency defibrillation is indicated for acute ventricular fibrillation or ventricular tachycardia with no audible or palpable pulse; it is ineffective for asystole or pulseless electrical activity. Defibrillation delivers an electrical discharge through paddles or pads applied to both sides of the chest. Automated external defibrillators (AEDs) are frequently used by first responders although manual defibrillators require less downtime from CPR. Procedure:

- Turn on the AED.
- Apply pads to chest (position may vary according to manufacturer). For infants and small children, if pads touch when applied in the directed positions for an adult, apply one to chest and one to back.
- Plug in the connector if necessary.
- Do not touch the patient while the AED analyzes heart rhythm.

- Follow directions for shocking (or resuming CPR if rhythm is not shockable) and warn others to stand clear.
- Continue CPR beginning with compressions immediately after shock is delivered for 2 minutes or 5 cycles between defibrillations.

If the patient is wet, wipe off the chest before applying pads. Remove any transdermal patches on the chest, and shave excessive hair before applying pads. If the patient has an implanted device, the pads should be placed at least 1 in (2.5 cm) away.

SPECIAL ARRESTS AND PERI-ARREST SITUATIONS

Special arrests and peri-arrest situations include:

- **Drowning**: For water rescue, start with ventilation because compressions are ineffective. On land, open the patient's airway and check for breathing (respiratory arrest may occur before cardiac arrest). If there are no respirations, ventilate twice and check his or her pulse. If there is no pulse, begin CPR at a 30:2 ratio and defibrillate as soon as possible for VT/VF or follow asystole protocol, depending on the situation. If the patient vomits (common), turn him or her to one side, clear the mouth/suction, and resume CPR.
- **Electrical shock or lightning**: Begin CPR following standard protocol. Early intubation may be necessary if face, mouth, or neck burns are present. Maintain spinal stabilization because of the risk of back/neck injury. Provide an IV access line and fluids for extensive tissue injury after resuscitation.
- **Pregnancy**: Begin CPR following standard protocol. If the fundus height is at or above the umbilicus, use lateral uterine displacement (LUD) during CPR to relieve aortocaval compression. Alert resources for immediate peri-mortem C-section (in the second half of a pregnancy) if ROSC is not achievable or resuscitation is futile.
- **Hypothermia**: If no pulse or respiration is detectable, begin immediate CPR (30:20) and defibrillate as soon as possible. Remove any wet clothing (during resuscitation if possible) and begin with warming protocols. Manage the patient's airway/ventilation/oxygen supplementation with warm, humidified oxygen. After ROSC, warm the patient to 32-34 °C. Treat the underlying cause, such as drug overdose. Do not consider terminating efforts until the patient is rewarmed.
- **Electrolyte imbalance**: Sodium, magnesium (except for extreme hypermagnesemia), and calcium abnormalities rarely lead to cardiac arrest. However, hyperkalemia (high potassium) (>6.5 mEq/L/mmol/L) may be lethal. Stabilize the heart cells with 5-10 mL of 10% calcium chloride or 10-20 mL of 10% calcium gluconate; shift potassium to the cells with 1 mEq/kg sodium bicarbonate and 25 g 50% glucose (unless he or she is hyperglycemic) with 10 U regular insulin (if available, to prevent hyperglycemia) and 2.5 mg albuterol (per nebulizer); and provide diuresis with 20-40 mg furosemide (per protocol).
- **Trauma**: Follow standard protocol, but the patient may require cervical spine stabilization and advanced airway/ventilation or cricothyrotomy, depending on the injuries. Use barriers to protect yourself from blood. Note: A chest blow may cause VF, requiring rapid defibrillation.

POST-RESUSCITATION RETURN OF SPONTANEOUS CIRCULATION (ROSC)

If a patient undergoing resuscitation has **return of spontaneous circulation (ROSC)**, his or her ventilation and oxygenation must be supported to maintain the oxygen saturation ≥94% but less than 100% to avoid hyperoxia. Ventilation should be maintained at 10-12 breaths per minute with an ETCO$_2$ value at 35-40 mmHg. Hyperventilation must be avoided. Hypotension (systolic BP <90 mmHg) should be treated with an IV bolus (1-2 L saline) and vasopressor infusion. Treatable causes (the five H's and five T's) should be addressed, and a 12-lead ECG should be used to monitor the patient's condition. If the patient is nonresponsive, therapeutic hypothermia (to 32-34 °C) for 12-24 hours may be considered as a neuroprotective measure. If the patient is responsive and able to follow commands, he or she should be immediately transported to the appropriate receiving facility: the ICU or cardiac cath lab for acute myocardial infarction (AMI) or ST-elevated myocardial infarction (STEMI) for percutaneous coronary intervention (PCI). Note: Brain damage begins within 4-6 minutes of cardiac arrest, and it is irreversible after 8-10 minutes.

TERMINATION OF RESUSCITATION EFFORTS

Criteria for termination of resuscitation efforts include the following considerations:

- ≥18 years
- Arrest is cardiac-related and not a condition that may respond to hospital treatment
- Endotracheal intubation was successful and maintained throughout resuscitation efforts
- Standard advanced cardiac life support efforts were used
- Resuscitation efforts maintained for 25 minutes or asystole through four rounds of drugs
- At the time of the decision to terminate, the patient exhibits asystole or an agonal rhythm (the bizarre, ineffective, wide ventricular rhythm associated with dying)
- Official DNR order
- Newborn: No heartbeat detected after 10 minutes of CPR

Note: Older age, quality of life, and time of collapse prior to EMS arrival are not criteria for termination. Generally, resuscitation efforts are continued until arrival at the receiving facility on those patients younger than 18 unless the child has a terminal disease and an advance directive that limits resuscitation efforts. Prior to termination, the EMS provider should have direct communication with medical oversight and consult/advise the family members that are present. Family resistance must be noted and reported. Criteria for withholding resuscitation include DNR status, obvious signs of death (such as rigor mortis/lividity), or conditions that are unsafe for the rescuer.

WITHHOLDING RESUSCITATION ATTEMPTS

Although the goal of EMS is to save lives, it is not always possible or ethical to carry out resuscitation efforts. **Withholding resuscitation** is justified under the following conditions:

- The patient's condition is not compatible with life (massive injuries, decapitation, crushed chest, severe open head injury with loss of brain tissue), and the patient is not breathing and has no pulse.
- The patient exhibits obvious signs of death, such as rigor mortis or livor mortis, indicating that he or she can no longer be resuscitated.
- The patient has a do-not-resuscitate (DNR) form available, and it is properly signed. Note: The EMS provider cannot accept the word of family or friends that the patient does not want to be resuscitated without a DNR order.
- Conditions are unsafe to approach the patient and/or administer resuscitation efforts. This may occur, for example, if there are gunshots heard in the area, if the patient is pinned under a motor vehicle, or if the patient cannot safely be reached in time because of difficult terrain.

CPR Assistive Devices

Impedance Threshold Device (ITD)

The impedance threshold device (such as the ResQPOD ITD) is a small, single-use device that fits into the airway circuit (face mask or advanced airway) with CPR. During CPR, compressions generate both positive pressure that promotes cardiac output and, when released completely, negative pressure (a vacuum) within the thorax that refills the heart, so adequate negative pressure ensures better filling. During compressions with an ITD, a valve in the device allows air to escape, but, when the compressions are released, the valve closes to prevent the intake of air, increasing negative pressure and improving circulation on subsequent compressions; however, the device allows the EMS provider to ventilate the patient, and it has flashing timing lights every 6 seconds (so 1 ventilation with every flash equals 10 per minute). The ITD may double the blood flow to the heart and double the systolic BP as well as increase cerebral perfusion.

Automated Chest Compression Devices

With automated chest compression devices for CPR, manual CPR should be started while the equipment is obtained and readied. These devices are only intended for adults and nontraumatic arrests, and they must be removed for defibrillation.

- **Piston-driven device (Thumper)**: Uses pneumatic (air) power on a piston device set at a prescribed compression depth. The backboard must first be secured with straps, the device is slid into a slot in the backboard, the massager pad is placed over the sternum, the device is turned on, and the compression depth is then set. The device can also control ventilations and tidal volume.
- **LUCAS device**: It is also piston driven and is similar to the Thumper, but it applies decompression suction on recoil to increase negative pressure, and it does not provide for ventilations.
- **Load-distributing band/Vest CPR (AutoPulse)**: A device that contains a backboard and fits like a vest around the patient's chest and applies compression to the chest and around the thorax, increasing perfusion pressure. It can be set for continuous compressions or 30:2, and it automatically adjusts to the patient's size.

Trauma

Trauma Overview

BLUNT TRAUMA

Blunt trauma can be the result of a variety of accidents/injuries:

- **Motor vehicle crashes**: Result in 30–40% of accidental deaths and half of closed-head and spinal cord injuries with injuries usually more serious with ejection, lateral (T-bone) impacts, and unrestrained patients, although lap belts increase the risk of abdominal injury (bowel injury in children). Shoulder belts may cause vascular injuries. Injuries include crush (compression), shear (tearing), and burst (rupture from sudden increase in pressure). The risk of death increases if another vehicle occupant dies. Most frontal collisions result in injuries from impact with the steering wheel, dashboard, windshield, or floorboards. More severe injuries occur at speeds of >25 mph.
- **Motorcycle crashes**: Approximately 75% of deaths are from head injuries, but injuries to the spine, pelvis, and extremities, including limb loss, are common.
- **Pedestrian and motor vehicle impacts**: Often results in Waddell's triad (tibiofibular or femur fracture, trunk injury, and head/face injury). Small children are often run over, and adults are thrown over the car by the impact. Intra-abdominal injury and pelvic fractures may occur from fender contact with the hips.
- **Falls**: The most common cause of accidental death in geriatric patients is by falling. Anticoagulants increase the risk of injury with falls. The degree of injury depends on the patient's weight and the fall distance. Injuries are most severe with a fall distance of >20 feet for adults and >10 feet for children. A three-story fall results in 50% mortality; the mortality is almost 100% for five-story falls. Horizontal landings cause fewer injuries (hand, wrist, head/face, and abdominal) than feet-first landings, which often result in fractures of the heel, leg, pelvis, and/or vertebrae.
- **Sports injuries/Play**: Injuries vary depending on the type of injury but can include head injuries, musculoskeletal injuries, and abdominal injuries. Helmet or knee contact to the flank area may cause kidney injury. The most common injuries are strains, sprains, and knee injuries.
- **Assaults**: Assaults are most common in young males and include facial and head injuries. Severe torso injuries may occur with kicking/stomping. If the patient is intoxicated and has altered consciousness, then he or she is treated as having a head injury. Assaults include domestic violence and child abuse, with distinctive patterns of injury.

PENETRATING TRAUMA

Penetrating traumas are most often the result of violence, such as gunshot wounds and puncture wounds.

- **Gunshot wounds**: Solid organs (brain, liver, spleen) often suffer more damage than more elastic tissues (fat, lungs). If a bullet is not deformed after entering the tissue, it tends to tumble (180°), creating a tunnel of injury (permanent cavity) and damage to the surrounding tissue (temporary cavity). If the bullet is deformed, it causes more severe localized tissue damage. Bullets usually have a straight trajectory, but they may be deflected if they strike bone. Shotgun blasts within 15 feet cause more damage than other gunshot wounds, but they are usually less severe at a distance.
- **Puncture wounds**:
  - *Stab:* Includes hand-driven objects (knives, glass shards, ice picks, or pieces of metal/wood). Surface puncture wounds are often small, but their depth varies according to the instrument used, which should be removed surgically.
  - *Slash:* These are usually long but not deep lacerations.
  - *Impalement:* This usually results from objects larger than a knife, often from a fall onto an object, but it can include arrows and nails from pneumatic tools.

BLEEDING

IDENTIFYING TYPE AND SOURCE OF BLEEDING

Any type of trauma can induce bleeding, internal or external. Identifying the **type and source of bleeding** is critical in managing the bleed.

- **Arterial**: Bright-red spurting blood that is difficult to control; lessens as the BP falls
- **Venous**: Dark-red blood flowing in a steady stream; may be copious, but is easier to control than an arterial bleed
- **Capillary**: Oozing; usually clots spontaneously
- **Internal**: Usually evidenced by increasing signs of shock or discolored swollen, painful tissue, guarding, coughing up blood, or rectal bleeding. Long-bone fractures (femur) and pelvic fractures may result in severe blood loss.

Prehospital Interventions: Using standard precautions and PPE as indicated, apply sterile gauze dressing and pressure with the fingertips if it is a small bleed or apply direct hand pressure if it is more copious. As dressings saturate, add new dressings but don't remove the old ones. A tourniquet may be needed if the bleeding is uncontrolled. Maintain the patient in the shock position, especially with an arterial bleed or severe blood loss, and keep him or her warm. Avoid giving food or fluids, and transport immediately for severe bleeding. Severity relates to the rate of blood loss volume and the age and health of patient. The blood volume is less with pediatric patients. Moving the injured area, a change in body temperature, medications, and the removal of bandages may impair clotting.

CONTROLLING VISIBLE HEMORRHAGE

Many types of hemorrhage exist, but hemorrhage in the general sense means severe bleeding or significant loss of blood. When the source of a patient's blood loss can be visualized, there are ways to control the hemorrhage. First and foremost, the patient's airway, breathing, and circulation should be assessed. Once those have been evaluated, the hemorrhage site should be freed from constrictive clothing or attire of any kind so that the site is exposed. In cases of minor bleeding, direct pressure should be applied to the injury site to stop the bleeding, the site should be cleansed with soap and water, and a sterile dressing should be applied. In cases of serious hemorrhage, the risks of causing further damage to an injured site should be considered against the possible benefits of applying direct pressure to the area.

TOURNIQUETS

Tourniquets are recommended as life-saving devices for uncontrolled arterial hemorrhage of the extremities that cannot be controlled with pressure or other means. The types of trauma tourniquets that are recommended were developed by the military but are now in common use for emergency care. The Combat Application Tourniquet (CAT) and the SOF Tactical Tourniquet (SOF-T) are adjustable bands with a windlass stick to tighten and a windlass clip and strap. The tourniquet is applied about 2 inches above the wound or above the knee for lower leg wounds and above the elbow for lower arm wounds. After the tourniquet is applied, the windlass is twisted to tighten until the distal pulse disappears and bleeding slows considerably or stops. Once bleeding is controlled, the windlass is secured. The tourniquet should be kept open to the field of vision so it is constantly monitored. If no tourniquet is available, a BP cuff can be applied and inflated.

REVISED TRAUMA SCORE (RTS) AND PRIMARY ASSESSMENT OF TRAUMA PATIENTS

The revised trauma score (RTS) uses the Glasgow Coma Scale (GCS) score, systolic BP, and respiration rate to establish a score for triage. A score of 0-4 is assigned for each category:

	GCS Score	Systolic BP	Respirations
4	13-15	90+	10-29
3	9-12	76-89	30+
2	6-8	50-75	6-9
1	4-5	1-49	1-5
0	3	0	0

For triage purposes, an RTS of 12 indicates delayed treatment; 11 indicates urgent, and a score of 3-10 indicates that immediate treatment is required. A score of less than 3 indicates death or an unsurvivable condition.

In the hospital setting, the RTS is further interpreted using a weighted scale for more accuracy in predicting survival. The scores (0-4) are combined using a weighting formula: RTS = $(0.9368 \times$ GCS score) + $(0.7326 \times$ BP score) + $(0.2908 \times$ RR score). Thus, an RTS can range from 0 to 7.84.

Primary assessment of trauma patients should include evaluation of the airway, breathing, and circulation (including observing for deviated septum, changes in chest wall motion, fractures, sucking chest wounds, and crepitation [of the neck and chest] from air), as well as an assessment of disability with a brief neurological exam (pupils, limb movement) and GSC/RTS. Removing the patient's clothing for examination and logrolling him or her are part of the assessment.

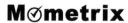

ISSUES OF TRANSPORT MODE AND DESTINATION

Issues that arise surrounding transport modes and destination when handling trauma include:

- Patient's triage status and duration of time needed for transport
- Distance from receiving institution
- Patient's need for specialized equipment or medical specialists and availability in ambulance and at receiving institution
- Airlift vs ambulance transport for critically ill
- Low acuity patient's insistence on transport to hospital when transport is deemed unnecessary
- Patient refusal to be transported to hospital
- Patient incompetent to make decisions about transport or unconscious and unable to make decisions
- Use of lights or sirens continuously, intermittently, or not at all (Lights-only may be used to minimize patient's anxiety and to reduce distractions for EMS. Sirens may be used intermittently at intersections and when traffic congestion is slowing progress.)
- Patient dies prior to transportation
- Patient dies en route (Regulations may vary by state and jurisdiction but may require the ambulance to wait for the medical examiner.)

Chest Trauma

CHEST WOUNDS

Chest wounds can be characterized as sucking wounds or impalements.

- **Sucking**: This is an open pneumothorax in which air is sucked into the thoracic cavity, deflating the lung, usually through a penny-size or larger wound. Patients will exhibit respiratory distress, absent breath sounds on the affected side, wound gurgling on inspiration, and bubbling of blood around the wound. Prehospital Interventions: Apply an occlusive dressing with an Asherman Chest Seal dressing or with Vaseline gauze covered with secured (taped on three sides) plastic wrap or aluminum foil and place the patient in a position of comfort.
- **Impalement**: This is a penetrating wound with an object impaled into the chest. Symptoms may be similar to those listed above, depending on the site of impalement and the depth. Impalement may cause hemothorax, tension pneumothorax, or pericardial tamponade. Prehospital Interventions: Expose the wound area, and secure the object manually with a bulky dressing. Do not remove the object unless it is necessary for performing chest compressions (CPR). Control any bleeding.

FRACTURED RIBS AND FLAIL CHEST

Fractured ribs usually result from severe blunt trauma (motor vehicle accident, physical abuse). Underlying injuries should be expected according to the area of fractures as follows:

- Upper two ribs: Injuries to the trachea, bronchi, or great vessels
- Right-sided ≥ rib 8: Liver trauma
- Left-sided ≥ rib 8: Spleen trauma

Pain may be the primary symptom of rib fractures, resulting in shallow breathing.

Flail chest (more common in adults and adolescents than children) occurs when at least three adjacent ribs are fractured, anteriorly and posteriorly, so that they float free of the rib cage. Variations include the sternum floating with ribs fractured on both sides. With flail chest, the chest wall cannot support changes in intrathoracic pressure, so paradoxical respirations occur with the flail area contracting on inspiration and expanding on expiration. Ventilation decreases.

Prehospital Interventions: Manage the patient's airway/ventilation/oxygen supplementation (PPV with BVM or intubation). Provide cardiac monitoring, an IV access line, and supportive care. Observe for signs of tension pneumothorax or hemothorax.

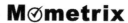

TENSION PNEUMOTHORAX

If not treated promptly, a sucking chest wound (open pneumothorax) may progress to a **tension pneumothorax,** especially if mechanical ventilation is used. A tension pneumothorax occurs when pressure in the pleural space exceeds that of the atmosphere, causing a mediastinal shift (which is usually difficult to assess visually) with displacement of the trachea away from the affected site, putting pressure against the great vessels (decreasing cardiac output), and putting pressure against the heart (resulting in tachycardia). Patients are usually in severe respiratory distress with jugular vein distension, absent breath sounds on the affected side, narrow pulse pressure, pulsus paradoxus, and unequal chest rise.

Prehospital Interventions: Place an airtight seal or Asherman Chest Seal over the open wound, manage the patient's airway/ventilation/oxygen supplementation to an oxygen saturation level of ≥94%, provide cardiac monitoring, start an IV access line, and provide rapid transport. Tension pneumothorax will require needle decompression or insertion of a chest tube (according to protocol).

HEMOTHORAX

Hemothorax occurs with bleeding into the pleural space, usually from major vascular injury such as tears in the intercostal vessels, lacerations of the great vessels, or trauma to the lung tissue. Hemothorax is most common with penetrating wounds. A small bleed may be self-limiting and seal, but a tear in a large vessel can result in massive bleeding, followed quickly by hypovolemic shock from decreased circulating blood. The pressure from the blood may result in the inability of the lung to ventilate and a mediastinal shift. Clots in the chest area may trigger fibrinolysis, which breaks down clots and increases bleeding. Often a hemothorax occurs with a pneumothorax, especially in severe chest trauma. Further symptoms include severe respiratory distress, decreased breath sounds, unequal breath sounds, dullness on auscultation, jugular venous distension, and shock.

Prehospital Interventions: Manage the patient's airway/ventilation/oxygen supplementation, provide an IV access line and fluid bolus for shock but avoid aggressive fluids because of the risk of hemodilution, provide the patient a position of comfort (the shock position if necessary), and provide rapid transport.

CARDIAC TAMPONADE

Cardiac tamponade occurs when fluid, usually blood, accumulates in the pericardial sac. If the fluid accumulates rapidly, the walls of the pericardial sac do not have time to stretch to accommodate the fluid, so the patient may quickly develop pulseless electrical activity (PEA) with fluid accumulation of 50-250 mL. If fluid accumulates slowly, such as with pericardial effusions associated with cancer, patients may tolerate up to 2 L of fluid before symptoms become acute. Cardiac tamponade compresses the heart and limits the venous return to the heart and blood flow into the ventricles, thereby reducing cardiac output. Symptoms: Beck's triad includes decreased arterial BP, increased jugular venous distension, and muffled heart sounds. Patients may be anxious, dyspneic, dizzy, and have angina-like pain.

Prehospital Interventions: Manage airway/high concentration oxygen, monitor the ECG, provide an IV access line and fluids as indicated, and provide rapid transport for pericardiocentesis.

> **Review Video: <u>Cardiac Tamponade</u>**
> Visit mometrix.com/academy and enter code: 920182

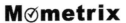

Abdominal and Genitourinary Trauma

ABDOMINAL AND GENITOURINARY ORGANS

The **peritoneum** lines the abdominal cavity. The anterior (front) area is the **intraperitoneal space**, which contains the stomach, the first part of the duodenum, the small intestines, and part of the large intestines and rectum as well as the liver, bile ducts, spleen, ovaries, part of the pancreas and ureters, and bladder. The posterior (back) **retroperitoneal space** contains part of the duodenum, the ascending and descending colon, and part of the rectum as well as part of the pancreas and ureters, the kidneys, the adrenal glands, the uterus, and the fallopian tubes. The ovaries, uterus, and fallopian tubes comprise the female reproductive system. **Solid organs** include the liver, spleen, ovaries, uterus, pancreas, kidneys, and adrenals. **Hollow organs** include the bile ducts, stomach, large and small intestines, fallopian tubes, ureters, and bladder.

EVISCERATIONS AND IMPALED OBJECTS

Eviscerations occur with open abdominal wounds, such as opening incisions or traumatic injuries, which allow the internal organs (often the intestines) to protrude externally. Surgical repair is required to reinsert the organs into the abdomen. The patient may go into shock, especially if the evisceration is part of other major injuries (common in trauma cases).

Prehospital Interventions: Provide supportive care; cover the eviscerated organs with thick, sterile gauze dressings moistened with NS, but do not attempt to reinsert them, manage the patient's airway/ventilation/oxygen supplementation as needed, and provide rapid transport.

Impalements occur when an object penetrates the abdomen and remains in place and may be associated with multiple internal injuries and bleeding.

Prehospital Interventions: Do not remove the object, but do expose the abdomen and manually secure the object with bulky dressings and control any bleeding. Provide supportive care, manage the patient's airway/ventilation/oxygen supplementation as needed, and provide rapid transport.

BLUNT ABDOMINAL WOUNDS

Abdominal trauma may result in **blunt wounds**, which may occur as the result of motor vehicle accidents, motorcycle accidents, pedestrian injuries, sports injuries, falls, blast injuries, and assaults. Blunt injuries comprise crush (compression), shear (tearing), and burst (sudden increased pressure) injuries. Motor vehicle accidents often result in liver injury in the passenger with impact on that side of the vehicle and spleen injury in the driver with impact on the driver's side. Other injuries from blunt trauma include damage to the diaphragm, retroperitoneal hematomas, and intestinal injuries, including perforation. Symptoms of internal injuries include pain, guarding, abdominal distension, discoloration, tenderness on movement, and evidence of lower rib fractures. Some patients may exhibit rectal bleeding and/or vomiting of blood.

Prehospital Interventions: Provide airway/ventilation/oxygen supplementation as needed, place in a position of comfort, treat for shock if indicated (especially with suspected internal bleeding), and provide rapid transport for patients in an unstable condition.

PENETRATING ABDOMINAL WOUNDS

Abdominal trauma may result in **penetrating wounds**, which are almost always related to gunshot wounds (high energy), shotgun wounds (medium energy), or knife wounds (low energy). Gunshot and shotgun wounds tend to cause more extensive damage than stab wounds, especially to the colon, liver, spleen, and diaphragm, and they may have an exit wound. Interior injuries may be extensive because the bullet damages tissues and may ricochet off of bone. Hemorrhage and peritonitis (especially with perforation of the intestines) are common complications. Pain is often more acute with injury to hollow organs than to solid organs, although blood loss may be severe with injury to the liver, spleen, or kidneys, and blood collecting in the retroperitoneal space may not be evident on inspection, palpation, or auscultation.

Prehospital Interventions: Control external bleeding, manage the patient's airway/ventilation/oxygen supplementation, mobilize the spine if indicated, and apply a pneumatic antishock garment (PASG) if indicated for shock or pelvic fracture (contraindicated with difficulty breathing, pregnancy [second and third trimesters], evisceration, an impaled object, and open fractures).

HEPATIC (LIVER) INJURY

Hepatic (liver) injury is the most common cause of death (mortality rates of 8–25%) from abdominal trauma and is often associated with multiple organ damage, so symptoms may be nonspecific. **Liver injuries** are classified according to the degree of injury, as follows:

I. Tears in the capsule with hematoma
II. Laceration(s) of the parenchyma (<3 cm)
III. Laceration(s) of the parenchyma (>3 cm)
IV. Destruction of 25–75% of a lobe from burst injury
V. Destruction of >75% of a lobe from burst injury
VI. Avulsion (tearing away)

Hemorrhage is a common complication of hepatic injury. Treatment often includes intravenous fluids for fluid volume deficit as well as blood products (plasma, platelets) for coagulopathies.

Prehospital Interventions: Manage the patient's airway/ventilation/oxygen supplementation, control external bleeding, treat signs of shock, start an IV access line with fluid bolus if indicated (but beware of hemodilution), provide rapid transport for an unstable patient.

SPLENIC INJURY

The spleen is the most frequently injured solid organ in blunt trauma because it's not well protected by the rib cage and it is very vascular. Symptoms may be very nonspecific. Kehr's sign (radiating pain in the left shoulder) indicates intra-abdominal bleeding, and Cullen's sign (ecchymosis around the umbilicus) indicates hemorrhage from a ruptured spleen. Some may have right upper abdominal pain, although diffuse abdominal pain often occurs with blood loss, associated with hypotension. **Splenic injuries** are classified according to the degree of injury, as follows:

- Tear in splenic capsules or hematoma
- Laceration of parenchyma (<3 cm)
- Laceration of parenchyma (>3cm)
- Multiple lacerations of parenchyma or burst-type injury

Treatment may be supportive if the injury is not severe; otherwise, suturing or removal of the spleen may be needed.

Prehospital Interventions: Control external bleeding, manage the patient's airway/ventilation/oxygen supplementation, treat signs of shock, start an IV access line with fluid bolus if indicated (but beware of hemodilution), and provide rapid transport for an unstable patient.

TRAUMATIC INJURIES TO GENITALIA

PENIS

- Blunt, penetrating, crushing, or amputating injuries as well as urethral penetration. Pain and bleeding may be severe.
- **Prehospital Interventions**: Control external bleeding, do not removed the impaled object. Provide pain management, an ice pack to reduce swelling, and emotional support.

SCROTUM

- Blunt, penetrating, or crushing injury may result in severe pain and swelling.
- **Prehospital Interventions**: As above but do not attempt to relieve scrotal pressure except with ice packs.

VAGINA

- May have external bruising and tearing (especially with sexual assault) at the vaginal opening. There may be pain, swelling, and bleeding.
- **Prehospital Interventions**: Control external bleeding, and provide emotional support, but do not remove impaled objects.

VULVA

- May include blunt, penetrating, or crushing injury as well as bite marks (with sexual assault) with pain, swelling, and bleeding.
- **Prehospital Interventions**: As above. Report sexual assaults according to protocol.

Orthopedic Trauma

MUSCULOSKELETAL SYSTEM

The musculoskeletal system includes 206 bones including long bones (e.g., the femur in the thigh), short bones (e.g., the carpal bones in the fingers), and flat bones (e.g., the sternum). The outer hard shell of the bone is the cortex, and the inner porous area is the trabecular bone. The vertebrae lack the cortex layer. Long bones have three parts: The middle section is the diaphysis, followed by the metaphyses, and then the epiphyses (the bone ends). In growing children, an epiphyseal plate of cartilage separates the metaphyses and epiphyses, allowing bone growth. This closes in adults, but damage to this area in a child may impair bone growth. The middle part of the short bones contains yellow bone marrow (fatty tissue). Red bone marrow, which produces blood cells, is found in the middle of the flat bones (pelvis, sternum, ribs, and scapula) and at the ends (epiphyses) of long bones. The skeletal system is connected by cartilage and tendons, and it is protected, supported, and allowed movement by about 700 soft-tissue muscles.

> **Review Video: Muscular System**
> Visit mometrix.com/academy and enter code: 967216
>
> **Review Video: Skeletal System**
> Visit mometrix.com/academy and enter code: 256447

ASSESSMENT OF MUSCULOSKELETAL INJURIES

Assessment of musculoskeletal injuries should include the following:

- Palpation/inspection for tissue damage, swelling, deformity, and tenderness
- Comparison with the opposite side if a limb is involved
- Assessment of neurovascular status (pulse, color, sensation, and function) distal to (below) the fracture
- Assessment of the six P's:
  - **Pain** (site of pain, degree, character)
  - **Pallor** (below the fracture or generalized)
  - **Paresthesia** (impaired sensation below fracture)
  - Distal **pulses** (intact, weak, absent)
  - **Paralysis** (with or without impaired sensation)
  - **Pressure** (often associated with swelling and pain)
- Assessment of age and general condition (geriatric patients are more likely to have fractures from relatively minor injuries because of osteoporosis)

If a fracture or dislocation is suspected, then the area should be splinted or immobilized for transport. Types of splints include rigid (should be padded), nonrigid (moldable), traction, air (pneumatic devices), pillow/blanket, short spine board, and long spine board. Splinting procedures are similar for adults, pediatric patients, and geriatric patients.

FRACTURES

Fractures usually result from trauma (falls, auto accidents), but **pathologic (nontraumatic) fractures** can result from minor force to diseased bones (osteoporosis or cancerous lesions). **Stress fractures** are caused by repetitive trauma (forced marching). **Salter-Harris fractures** involve the cartilaginous epiphyseal plate near the ends of long bones in children who are growing, and this can impair bone growth. Fractures can be classified as open or closed:

- **Open fractures** have soft-tissue injury and a break in the skin overlying the fracture, including puncture wounds from external forces or bone fragments; these can result in osteomyelitis (bone infection).
- **Closed fractures** involve a broken bone but no break in the skin.

Symptoms include pain, deformity or angulation, swelling, bruising, inability to move the joint or bear weight, grating on movement, and impaired function or circulation. Isolated fractures are usually not life threatening, but pelvic and femur fractures may involve severe blood loss.

Prehospital Interventions: Cover open wounds with sterile dressings, manually stabilize and immobilize the fracture area, but do not replace protruding bones, apply a cold pack, and place the patient in a position of comfort.

NONTRAUMATIC FRACTURES

Nontraumatic fractures occur when the bone weakens and can no longer support the body, such as may occur with a cancerous tumor of the bone or osteoporosis. Common fractures associated with osteoporosis include fractures of the vertebrae and hip. Osteoporotic fractures are most common in older adults, but they may also occur in adolescents with eating disorders. Infants and young children with multiple nontraumatic, non-abusive fractures may have a genetic disorder, such as osteogenesis imperfecta. Assessment of suspected fractures includes evaluating pain/tenderness, swelling around the fracture site, loss of sensation or movement, circulatory impairment (note the color of the skin, pallor or cyanosis), and deformity (especially noticeable in limb fractures).

Prehospital Interventions: Splint extremity fractures; manage the patient's airway/ventilation/oxygen supplementation as needed; and provide transport for treatment.

TYPES OF FRACTURES

Fractures can be classified by the location and style of the break.

Spiral: Common in toddlers who fall on an extended leg, breaking the tibia, but it may also occur with abuse in small children as a result of jerking on or twisting an extremity (usually the arm).

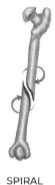

SPIRAL

Greenstick: Most common in children whose bones are less hard. It is usually quite painful but without deformity.

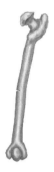

GREENSTICK

Displaced: Poses a risk of damage to surrounding tissues, including nerves and blood vessels and may lead to an open fracture if not properly splinted. The deformity is usually evident.

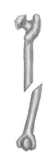

DISPLACED

Transverse: Usually occurs in long bones and is at risk of displacement unless it is splinted to prevent movement. Most often occurs from direct impact, such as sports injuries. May suggest abuse if occurring in small children.

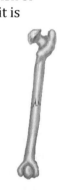

TRANSVERSE

Comminuted: Usually result from high-impact trauma, such as with motor vehicle accidents, and it is more common in older adults or those with weakened bones. This fracture is very painful and is often accompanied by swelling and muscle spasms.

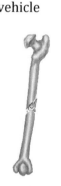

COMMINUTED

The femur is the long bone in the thigh. Although any part of the femur may fracture, fractures in the upper femur are common and are generally referred to as hip fractures. **Femur fractures** in young patients usually result from high-impact trauma, such as motor vehicle or pedestrian/motor vehicle accidents, whereas femur fractures in geriatric patients are most often from falls and are associated with osteoporosis. Patients may have many comorbidities and may present with dehydration and blood loss. Mortality rates for **hip fractures** are high, with 10% during the initial treatment and 25% over the next year. Symptoms of femur fractures include pain and deformity at the fracture site and an inability to walk or bear weight. A hematoma may be present.

Prehospital Interventions: Splint the leg in the position it was found in with a traction splint (Hare Traction Splint/Sager Emergency Traction Splint), flush open fractures with NS to remove debris, and apply an NS-moistened sterile gauze dressing, monitor vital signs and neurovascular status, and assess soft tissue for damage. Provide an IV access and fluids if indicated.

PREHOSPITAL MANAGEMENT OF FRACTURES

Prehospital management of fractures depends on the location and severity of the fracture:

- **Tibia/Fibula (lower leg)**: Manually immobilize during splinting. Splint the joint above and below the fracture(s) (upper thigh to ankle) with a padded rigid long-leg splint or a pneumatic splint, and then secure it to the other leg for additional support.
- **Shoulder**: Apply a sling to the affected side and secure the patient's arm against the body with a swathe to limit movement.
- **Knee**: If the pulse below the fracture is adequate and there is no deformity, splint with the knee straight. If there is deformity, splint the leg in the position it was found. If there is no pulse below the fracture, consult with medical assistance immediately. Never use a traction splint.
- **Clavicle (upper chest)**: Apply a sling to the affected side. (Common in young children who fall with an arm outstretched.)
- **Humerus (upper arm)**: Apply a sling to the affected side and swathe the arm to the body to limit movement.
- **Radius/Ulna (forearm)**: Splint from the elbow to the wrist and secure above and below the fracture. Elevate the arm.
- **Elbow**: Apply a sling to the affected side (often results from a fall).

AMPUTATIONS

Amputations may be partial or complete and result from crush, guillotine (cutting), or avulsion (twisting) injuries. A **simple amputation** requires no extrication and other injuries or shock are absent, but a **complex amputation** may involve multiple injuries, shock, and delayed treatment because of extrication. The amputated limb should be treated initially as though it could be reattached, although single digits (except the thumb) and lower limbs are not usually reattached. The part should be irrigated with normal saline (NS) to remove debris; wrapped in NS-moistened gauze; and placed in a sealed plastic bag, which should be immersed in ice water. The body part should not freeze and should not be placed directly on ice.

Prehospital Interventions: Manage the patient's airway/ventilation/oxygen supplementation; control bleeding by direct pressure or, if there is severe hemorrhage, by applying a BP cuff proximal to (above) the injury 70 mmHg greater than the systolic BP for <30 minutes. Irrigate the stump with NS if it is dirty, cover the open area with NS-moistened gauze, and elevate the stump.

PELVIC FRACTURES

Pelvic fractures represent about 3% of total fractures, but they pose a greater risk than most other types of fractures. **Pelvic fractures** most often result from a motor vehicle accident (50-60%) in adults and a pedestrian/motor vehicle impact (60-80%) in children. Pelvic fractures may be accompanied by major injuries to soft tissue and internal organs, especially the bladder, urethra (especially in children and women), and colon. A fracture on one side often results in a fracture on the other side as well. The primary cause of death after a pelvic fracture is hemorrhage with 50-70% of patients with unstable fractures requiring multiple transfusions. Geriatric patients have higher mortality rates than do younger patients. Symptoms include pain and tenderness, bloody urine, rectal bleeding, vaginal bleeding, retroperitoneal bleeding, hematoma over the fracture site, pain on hip motion, and signs of shock (with blood loss).

Prehospital Interventions: Monitor vital signs for indications of shock, position supine, apply PASG or a pelvic wrap device (per protocol) to stabilize and prevent excessive movement, and monitor the patient's airway, ventilation, and oxygen supplementation. Provide an IV access (large bore) and fluid as indicated.

PNEUMATIC ANTISHOCK GARMENT (PASG)

The pneumatic antishock garment (PASG) is indicated for hypovolemic shock and hypotension associated with and stabilization of pelvic and bilateral femur fractures. PASG is contraindicated with respiratory distress, pulmonary edema, pregnancy (second and third trimesters), heart failure, myocardial infarction, stroke, evisceration, abdominal or leg impalement, head injuries, and uncontrolled bleeding above the garment.

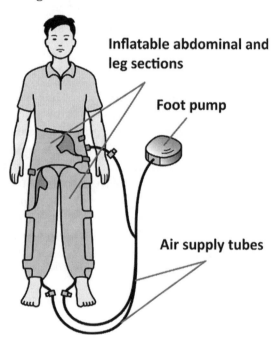

Inflatable abdominal and leg sections

Foot pump

Air supply tubes

The **procedure** for PASG use is as follows:

1. Place the garment flat on the patient-transport device/stretcher and transfer the patient onto the garment.
2. If the patient is already on the stretcher, place the garment under his or her legs first and then lift the patient's buttocks and slide the garment upward until the upper garment edge is 1 inch below the bottom ribs.
3. Secure the legs first and then the abdominal section with the Velcro straps. Attach the pump hoses to each leg and the abdominal section at the valves and close the stopcocks.
4. Open the stopcock for each leg and abdominal section one at a time, and inflate them one at a time.

After inflating each section, close the stopcock and check the vital signs. Stop inflating if the systolic BP ≥90 mmHg. If the systolic BP is still <90 mmHg, then proceed to filling the next section or sections until all three are filled.

FAT EMBOLISM

Fat embolism, a life-threatening complication of fractures, can occur when fat enters the venous circulatory system, typically lodging in the pulmonary microvasculature, causing increased pulmonary vascular resistance. Patients most at risk are the young with multiple injuries, the elderly, and those with preexisting disease (pulmonary hypertension, right ventricular disorder, or metastatic cancer). Preventive methods include stabilizing fractures of long bones or the pelvis within 24 hours of injury. Signs of fat embolism include abrupt bradycardia, hypertension, jugular venous distension, hypoxemia, decreased $ETCO_2$ concentration, chest and upper extremity petechiae, fat globules in the retina, and various cardiac irregularities such as dysrhythmias. As the pulmonary artery pressure increases, cardiac output decreases.

Prehospital Interventions: Immediate treatment includes 100% oxygen with mechanical ventilation per endotracheal tube with adequate IV fluids. Epinephrine or related drugs may be used for hemodynamic support per protocol.

JOINT DISLOCATIONS

Subluxation (partial dislocation of a joint) and **luxation** (complete dislocation of a joint) can cause neurovascular compromise, which can be permanent if reduction is delayed. This is especially a problem with **hip dislocations**, which most commonly occur in automobile accidents when the person's knees impact the dashboard. **Elbow dislocations** often result from athletic injuries and may cause nerve damage. **Shoulder dislocations** are the most common type and also often result from athletic injuries. They may become chronic. **Knee dislocations** may result in severe injury to the popliteal artery, and this can lead to amputation, so rapid transport and emergent surgical repair are indicated. Differentiating between fractures and dislocations can be difficult because the symptoms and appearance are often similar. A deformity may not be evident or may be obscured by edema, or edema may give the appearance of a deformity. Extensive bruising may occur with all types of injuries, and pain may occur even with minor soft-tissue injuries.

Prehospital Interventions: Splint and immobilize the area, and place the patient in a position of comfort.

SHOULDER INJURIES

A **sternoclavicular sprain** results from tearing of the ligaments that connect the sternum to the clavicle, usually resulting from a direct blow or twisting of an arm extended backward. Symptoms include pain near the top of the chest (below the neck). The pain increases on activity (such as lifting) and when lying on the affected side.

The **rotator cuff** comprises the muscle and ligaments of the shoulder joint. The bones in the joint include the scapula and humerus. Muscles (subscapularis, supraspinatus, infraspinatus, spines minor) and tendons anchor to the head of the humerus so that the arm can move in all directions, and ligaments connect the bones. Part of the rotator cuff is under the scapula. The most common injury to the rotator cuff is a tear in the supraspinatus tendon, so that the tendon is separated from its attachment, resulting from a violent pull on the arm, an abnormal rotation, or fall on an outstretched hand.

Prehospital Interventions: Provide a protective sling.

STRAINS AND SPRAINS

A **strain** is an overstretching of a part of the musculature ("pulled muscle") that causes microscopic tears in the muscle, usually resulting from excess stress or overuse of the muscle. The onset of pain is usually sudden with local tenderness on use of the muscle. A **sprain** is damage to a joint, with a partial rupture of the supporting ligaments and/or tendons, usually caused by wrenching or twisting that may occur with a fall. The rupture can damage blood vessels, resulting in edema, tenderness at the joint, and pain on movement with pain increasing over 2–3 hours after the injury. An avulsion fracture (the bone fragment is pulled away by a ligament) may occur with strain.

Prehospital Interventions: Immobilize the area for transport, use rest, ice, compression, and elevation (the RICE protocol), and monitor the patient's neurovascular status (especially for sprains) by checking the pulse, capillary refill, color, and sensation distal to (below) the injury.

SPLINTING AND SPINAL MOTION RESTRICTION
LONG SPINAL BOARD AND SPLINTING BY TRACTION

Various methods of splinting and spinal motion restriction should be considered by the emergency medical responder, based on the patient's method of injury and symptoms:

- **Long spinal board**: If spinal injury is suspected, place a cervical collar on the patient before placing the patient on the long board. With one person stabilizing the head and neck, the patient is logrolled onto one side and the board is positioned against the patient so that the patient can be logrolled back onto the board. Once the patient is positioned on the board, padding such as rolled towels should be placed about the head, neck, and shoulders to provide further support and to ensure the head remains in a neutral position. The patient is secured by straps.
- **Splinting by traction**: Assess patient for signs/symptoms of mid-shaft femur fracture without lower leg or hip injury. Ask partner to apply the ankle hitch and apply manual traction and then to elevate the leg. Slide the long-leg device under the leg and secure with the ischial strap by the hip. Fasten the ankle hitch to the device and apply traction according to manufacturer's guidelines until the patient feels some relief of discomfort. Secure the rest of the leg with straps. Reassess circulation, sensation, and motor function. Place patient on a long spinal board and secure the patient and the device to the long board.

SEATED SPINAL MOTION RESTRICTION USING THE KENDRICK EXTRICATION DEVICE

Seated spinal motion restriction (SMR) using the Kendrick Extrication Device (KED) is indicated for a seated patient who is unable to self-extricate, is conscious and stable, and complains of head, neck, or back pain. Ask another person to continually stabilize the patient's head from behind and then check the patient's hands and feet for sensation and movement:

1. Apply cervical collar. Support the chest and lean the patient forward ≤45 degrees and place the KED in position behind the patient.
2. Move the patient back to upright position and fasten the straps (usually color coded) across the abdomen first and then the chest. Before fastening the chest strap, ask the patient to take a deep breath to ensure the strap doesn't restrict breathing.
3. Then fasten leg straps by bringing each strap under the buttocks and up between the legs and then to the side to fasten. Male patients may need to adjust their genitals.
4. Last make sure the head contacts the padding of the device, bring the flaps about the sides of the face, and then apply the chin strap and the forehead strap.
5. Check sensations and movement in the hands and feet again and then move the patient onto a long board and then onto a stretcher.
6. Remove KED but leave the cervical collar in place.

Soft Tissue Trauma

OPEN SOFT-TISSUE INJURIES

Injury	Characteristics	Prehospital Interventions
Abrasion	Painful superficial scraping of the outermost layer of skin. There is little or no bleeding.	Irrigate with water or NS to remove debris and cover with nonadherent dressing.
Laceration	A cut or break in the skin from impact with a sharp object. Bleeding may vary from mild to severe.	Apply pressure to control the bleeding, irrigate to remove debris if necessary, and cover with a dry sterile gauze dressing.
Puncture	Wound from impact with a sharp pointed object (knife, bullet); it may exhibit little external bleeding but major internal bleeding and soft-tissue damage. An exit wound may be present.	Apply pressure to control any bleeding, manage the patient's airway/ventilation/oxygen supplementation, and provide rapid transport if the patient's condition is unstable.
Impaled object	Penetrating object remains in wound.	Leave the object in place and pad with bulky dressings.
Foreign body in eye(s)	Patient has pain, tearing, redness, and blurred or impaired vision from dirt, dust, chemicals, or other materials in the eye(s).	Cover both eyes loosely (avoiding pressure) to prevent movement. If it is chemical contamination, flush the eye(s) with copious amounts of NS or water.
Avulsions	The skin and underlying soft tissue are torn away, such as with a degloving injury, from any part of the body, although lower extremity injury is the most common. Bleeding may be severe, especially if vessels are torn or exposed.	Flush with sterile water or NS to remove debris if necessary, apply pressure and dressings to control bleeding and protect tissue, apply an ice pack, seal the avulsed skin and tissue in a plastic bag, and place in ice water for possible reimplantation or skin grafts. Return loose flaps to their anatomic positions.
Blast injury	Involves varying degrees of soft-tissue injury and sometimes amputations, fractures, impalements, traumatic brain injuries, ruptured eardrum, pulmonary injury, perforated bowel, and burns.	Manage the patient's airway/ventilation/oxygen supplementation, control bleeding and shock, provide CPR if necessary, supportive care, and rapid transport.

CLOSED SOFT TISSUE INJURIES

Injury	Characteristics	Prehospital Interventions
Contusion	Results from blunt or compressive pressure to a muscle and is a common sports injury. These may include other injuries, such as sprains, strains, fractures, and damage to internal organs. Symptoms include tenderness, pain on movement, and bruising. If bruising is in the shape of an instrument, it usually indicates abuse.	Provide RICE therapy and supportive care.
Hematoma	Collection of blood within the tissue because of damaged blood vessels from injury, underlying fracture, or medications (such as warfarin). These may be small or very large, and patients may lose ≥1 L of blood. Symptoms may include pain and swelling.	Provide supportive care for small contusions (which often resolve spontaneously), RICE therapy, and monitor for signs of continued bleeding.
Crush injury	External pressure may cause severe internal injuries, such as fractures and organ rupture.	Manage the patient's airway, ventilation, oxygen supplementation, and shock as needed, control bleeding, and provide supportive care.

CLASSIFICATION OF BURNS AND RULE OF NINES

Burn injuries may be chemical, electrical, or thermal and are assessed by the area affected, percentage of the body burned, and the depth of the burn, as follows:

- **First-degree burns** are superficial and affect the epidermis, causing erythema and pain.
- **Second-degree burns** extend through the dermis (partial thickness), resulting in blistering and sloughing of the epidermis and severe pain.
- **Third-degree burns** affect the underlying tissue, including the vasculature, muscles, and nerves (full thickness). Depending on the extent of the nerve damage, third-degree burns may present with less pain.

Burns are **classified** according to the American Burn Association's criteria as follows:

- **Minor**: <10% body surface area (BSA) or 2% BSA with third-degree burns without serious risk to the face, hands, feet, or perineum
- **Moderate**: 10–20% BSA combined second-degree and third-degree burns in adults; age <10 years or ≤10% third-degree without serious risk to the face, hands, feet, or perineum
- **Major**: ≥20% BSA; ≥10% third-degree burns; all burns are to the face, hands, feet, or perineum and will result in functional/cosmetic defect; or burns with inhalation or other major trauma

The **rule of nines** estimates the BSA burned:

- **Adults**: Head 9%, trunk (front) 18%, trunk (back) 18%, arm 9%, leg 18%, perineum 1%
- **Infants/Children**: Head 18%, trunk (front) 18%, trunk (back) 18%, arm 9%, leg 13.5%, perineum 1%

> **Review Video: Rule of Nines**
> Visit mometrix.com/academy and enter code: 846800

ELECTRICAL BURNS

Low-voltage **electrical contact** most often causes a localized burn (first to third degree) to the hand or mouth (toddlers) with various degrees of tissue damage, although mouth contact may also result in cardiac or respiratory arrest. High-voltage electrical contact results in an entry and an exit wound with internal damage occurring between these wounds. Electrical current takes the shortest route to leave the body (flowing along blood vessels and nerves), so if the current passes from hand to hand, damage is usually more severe than if it passes from a hand to a foot. Severe injury may result in damage to bones, compartment syndrome, organ failure, and cardiac arrest from asystole or ventricular fibrillation. Vessels may be mildly or severely damaged. Abdominal organs may be damaged. Neurological damage with unconsciousness is common, especially if the current passes through the head. Peripheral nerve damage is also common, and damage to the spinal cord may occur.

Prehospital Interventions: Manage the patient's airway, ventilation, and oxygen supplementation, provide CPR/defibrillation as needed, provide rapid transport (with the head elevated if it was involved), start an IV access line, and give fluid resuscitation if needed.

LIGHTNING BURNS AND INJURIES

Lightning injuries may occur with a direct strike (≤5%), side splash from a strike nearby, contact voltage when touching an item that has been struck, ground current (from a more distant strike), and blunt trauma from being too close to a strike (which often results in the patient being thrown). Symptoms may vary, but they can include external burns (Lichtenberg figures) in a fernlike pattern, acute pain, fixed and dilated pupils (temporary), eye injuries, confusion, headache, hearing loss, perforated eardrum, hypotension, paralysis/paresis, spinal cord injury, altered mental status, brain injury, fractures, and cardiac arrest. Patients may be responsive initially but lapse into unconsciousness as cerebral edema increases, resulting in secondary respiratory and/or cardiac arrest. Burns are usually mild because of the brief contact.

Prehospital Interventions: Manage the patient's airway, ventilation, and oxygen supplementation, provide CPR/defibrillation as needed, provide rapid transport (with the head elevated), start an IV access line, and give fluid resuscitation.

GENERAL MANAGEMENT OF CHEMICAL AND ELECTRICAL BURNS

Patients with severe burns may develop shock and impairment of all major body systems. If the burning process is ongoing, room-temperature water or NS should be applied to stop the burning and any smoldering clothes or jewelry should be removed, although if the clothing is adhered to the skin, it should be left in place. With facial or airway burns, the airway must be monitored constantly with interventions as necessary, and an IV access line should be provided for fluid replacement, based on the patient's weight and the extent of the burn (Parkland formula: 4 mL/kg/wt × BSA per 24 hours). The burned area should be covered with nonadherent dry clean dressings, and the patient should be kept warm for transport. Children experience greater fluid and heat loss because

74

of their greater body surface relative to their size, and the EMS provider should be alert to the possibility of child abuse. With **chemical burns**, any dry powder should be brushed off, and wet chemicals should be flushed with copious amounts of water (by a provider wearing gloves and eye protection). With **electrical burns**, internal burns may be more severe than external burns, and the patient is at risk of cardiac arrest.

DRESSINGS AND BANDAGES

Dressings and bandages may be appropriate when handling specific wounds or burns. Each type of dressing has specific characteristics meant to be used for specific purposes.

- **Sterile gauze**: 4×4 (sponge) or roller/wrapping gauze (Kerlix) used to protect skin or pack wounds to control bleeding. Roller gauze may be used to secure other dressings.
- **Nonadherent dressings**: Designed not to stick to open wounds because of their special coating (Teflon, foam, petrolatum, hydrogel). Used on abrasions, burns, and lightly draining wounds.
- **Occlusive dressings**: These have a waxy coating to make an air- and water-tight seal, but they are not as absorbent as gauze. Used for sucking chest wounds, abdominal eviscerations, and lacerations of the external jugular vein or carotid.
- **Trauma dressings**: Dressings that often include a nonadherent pad, a clotting agent embedded in the dressing, and an elastic wrap in one piece so that they can be rapidly applied (e.g., an ACE bandage), include QuikClot Combat Gauze and Celox Rapid hemostatic gauze. Especially useful to control bleeding and to apply pressure to a wound.
- **Adhesive, roller bandages**: May be elastic or nonelastic, and they are used to secure other dressings and/or apply compression.

CRUSH SYNDROME

Crush syndrome results from injury associated with crushing pressure to skeletal muscle from heavy weight, such as when trapped under falling debris for extended periods, especially more than four hours. Injuries include:

- Direct damage to cells
- Decreased circulation and impaired oxygenation of tissue, which cause leakage of cells and buildup of lactic acid
- Dying cells leak substances, such as toxins, proteins, and electrolytes, into surrounding tissue but remain localized because of pressure
- With release of pressure, these substances enter general circulation:
  - *Potassium*: Causes cardiac dysrhythmias
  - *Myoglobin*: Damages kidneys
  - *Purines*: Damages lungs and liver

Symptoms vary depending on severity.

Prehospital Interventions: Assess airway, breathing, circulation, oxygen saturation, and VS. Provide oxygen at high concentration, establish IV access with NS infusion, monitor ECG for changes consistent with hyperkalemia. If hyperkalemia is evident, administer calcium chloride 500 mg IV over 2 minutes or administer aerosolized albuterol. Provide analgesia as indicated.

High-Pressure Injection

With high-pressure injection of substances, such as water, air, paint, kerosene, solvents, or oil, the substance travels until it meets resistance, such as from muscle or bone, and then spreads through the tissues. Injuries to the hand are most common. Damage may include dissection, damage to nerves, impaired oxygenation, tissue necrosis, bleeding into the tissues, and clot formation. Some substances may be toxic to cells, and the substance may be contaminated with bacteria. The injection site may be quite small and initial symptoms may be mild (pain, numbness) but pain and swelling tend to increase over time and can lead to compartment syndrome. Some substances may cause systemic symptoms (fever, elevated white blood cell count, and kidney damage).

Prehospital Interventions: Inspect, clean, and cover injection site. Provide analgesia as appropriate and elevate affected body part, assessing for signs of compartment syndrome (edema, tautness, severe pain and/or numbness, impaired circulation and sensation).

Traumatic Bites

Animal and Human Bite Wounds

Animal bites: Dog bites may cause any type of soft-tissue injury (lacerations, punctures, crush injury, avulsions) depending on the extent of the bite. Cat bites are often puncture bites with a high risk of infection. Pediatric and geriatric patients are most at risk of infection. Children are the most common victims of animal bites.

Prehospital Interventions: Check that the scene is safe and the animal is secured, control any bleeding, flush the wound with sterile NS or water, apply dressings, manage the patient's airway/ventilation/oxygen supplementation (especially with bites to the face/throat), and treat shock if needed. Check the rabies status of the animal involved if known. Report the bite according to legal requirements.

Human bites: If the bite is on the genitals, it indicates abuse. Most commonly bites are on the fingers from fist contact with someone's mouth. Human bites are prone to infection, especially if treatment is delayed.

Prehospital Interventions: Flush the wound with NS or water, apply a sterile dressing, and provide emotional support for victims of abuse. Document the patient's statement accurately in the event the bite becomes a legal matter.

Spider Bites

Certain spider bites can be lethal if not treated in a timely fashion:

Black Widow

Initially there are two faint fang marks with a pale area surrounded by a red-blue ring. Muscle cramps, pain radiating to the upper chest (arm bites) or abdomen (leg bites) and weakness within 2 hours increasing to generalized pain, headache, itching chills, nausea, vomiting, dyspnea, hypertension, cardiac abnormalities, shock, and coma.

Prehospital Interventions: Provide supportive care and analgesia and benzodiazepine to relieve muscle spasms (per protocol). Take the spider in a sealed plastic bag to the receiving facility.

BROWN RECLUSE

Red, swollen bite site with severe pain and itching; "red, white, and blue" sign (a pale center with a central blister and reddish-blue peripheral discoloration with the blister becoming ischemic and necrotic) leaving an open ulcerated area that covers with black eschar and may expand in size. The following systemic reactions may occur within 6–12 hours in some patients: fever, vomiting, jaundice, hypotension, change in mental status, hemolytic anemia, disseminated intravascular coagulation, renal failure, seizures, coma, and death.

Prehospital Interventions: Provide supportive care and analgesia. If symptoms are severe, provide an IV access line and fluids.

INSECT BITES AND STINGS

Insect bites should be treated by first identifying the insect (through the recognition of bite characteristics), and then treating as appropriate.

FIRE ANTS

Fire ant bites cause hives and blistering with severe itching, redness, pain, and burning. Some patients may develop systemic reactions and anaphylaxis.

Prehospital Interventions: Provide supportive care and cold compresses. Use the anaphylaxis protocol if necessary.

WASPS/BEES

Wasp and bee stings cause pain, itching, redness, and swelling (most common), but they may also cause severe allergic (hives) and/or anaphylactic (life-threatening) reactions.

Prehospital Interventions: Wipe the area with gauze or scrape it with a sharp instrument to remove the stinger, wash with soap and water, apply ice, and elevate. Give antihistamines for an allergic response. Use the anaphylaxis protocol if necessary.

TICKS

With tick bites, pain may occur at the bite site. Ticks carry numerous infections, including Lyme disease, so follow-up is essential.

Prehospital Interventions: Grasp the tick near the skin with tweezers and pull with steady upward pressure, disinfect the site, and save the tick in a plastic bag.

SCORPION STINGS

Scorpion stings typically cause local burning, itching, pain, and redness, and may cause severe neurologic or other systemic reactions, such as paresthesia, stroke, hypertension, tachycardia, respiratory distress, priapism, hemorrhage, nausea, and vomiting. Pregnant women may miscarry.

Prehospital Interventions: Immobilize the affected part below the level of the heart, apply cool compresses (the first 2 hours), monitor the patient's airway, ventilation, and oxygen supplementation, start an IV access and give fluids if needed, and administer norepinephrine for severe hypotension.

SNAKE BITES

Pit vipers include rattlesnakes, copperheads, and cottonmouths. They have erectile fangs that fold until they are aroused; their venom is primarily hemotoxic and cytotoxic, but it may also have neurotoxic properties (affecting the blood, cells, and nerves at the bite site and systemically). Symptoms vary depending on the amount of venom that is injected (many bites are dry).

- Wounds usually show one or two fang marks.
- Swelling may begin immediately, or it may be delayed for up to 6 hours.
- Pain may be severe.
- There may be a wide range of symptoms, including hypotension and impairment of blood clotting that can lead to excessive blood loss, depending upon the type and amount of venom.
- Progressive weakness, vision problems, nausea, vomiting, altered consciousness, and seizures are expected.

Prehospital Interventions: Note the time elapsed from the time of the bite to the time of transport, reassure the patient, immobilize the extremity, cleanse the wound with soap and water, apply an ice pack to slow venous return and reduce swelling, transport immediately for further treatment such as with antivenom, and mark the extent of the swelling on the skin every 15 minutes.

COMPLICATIONS ASSOCIATED WITH BURN INJURIES

Burn injuries begin with the skin but can affect all organs and body systems, especially with a major burn. Complications include the following:

- **Cardiovascular**: Cardiac output may fall by 50% as capillary permeability increases with vasodilation and fluid leaks from the tissues, resulting in hypovolemia and hypothermia. Vasoconstriction occurs as a compensatory mechanism, but it may impair circulation and result in further hypoxia.
- **Pulmonary**: Injury may result from smoke inhalation or (rarely) aspiration of hot liquid. Pulmonary injury is a leading cause of death from burns and is classified according to the degree of damage as follows:
    - **First**: Singed eyebrows and nasal hairs with possible soot in airways and slight edema, increasing hypoxia.
    - **Second**: Stridor, dyspnea, and tachypnea with edema and erythema of the upper airway, including the area of the vocal cords and epiglottis, resulting in severe hypoxia, sometimes with rapid onset.
- **Infection**: Open wounds are vulnerable to infection.
- **Circumferential burns**: Swelling beneath eschar can create a tourniquet effect, impairing distal circulation.

SKIN DAMAGE CAUSED BY RADIATION TREATMENT

Skin damage/burns caused by radiation treatment vary widely depending upon the dose, duration, fraction-size, treatment area, type of equipment, and condition of the patient. Acute radiation dermatitis usually occurs when radiation is higher than 10 Gy. Patients vary in the progression of symptoms. There may be an initial inflammatory response in the tissue, with increased perfusion and WBCs to the area.

STAGING OF SKIN DAMAGE

Acute skin damage begins within 2-3 weeks of exposure to radiation with changes that are reversible. Because the cells in the skin are constantly going through mitotic division, they are vulnerable to the effects of irradiation. Most reactions subside 1-3 months after therapy ends. Damage is staged according to the type and degree of reaction, and staging determines treatment:

- **Stage I**: Slight edema and inflammation with erythema that may result in burning, itching and discomfort, caused by dilation and increased permeability of capillaries
- **Stage II**: Dry, itching, scaly skin with partial sloughing of epidermis, caused by inability of basal epidermal cells to adequately replace surface cells and decreased functioning of skin glands.
- **Stage III**: Moist blistering skin with loss of epidermal tissue, serous drainage, and increased pain with exposure of nerves, caused by continued deterioration of skin.
- **Stage IV**: Loss of body hair and sweat gland suppression resulting in permanent hair loss, atrophy, pigment changes, and ulcerations, caused by accumulation of radiation in the tissues.

Head, Face, Neck, and Spine Trauma

ANATOMY OF THE BRAIN AND SPINAL CORD

The **brain** is protected by the skull and the meninges, the three layers of lining: the dura mater, arachnoid mater, and the pia mater. Brain tissue is comprised of gray matter (neurons [nerve cells]) and white matter (covered nerve pathways that conduct messages). The main part of the brain is the cerebrum, which is comprised of two hemispheres that contain the frontal parietal, temporal, and occipital lobes. The cerebrum controls higher brain functions, including thought, speech, vision, hearing, and action. The cerebellum lies in the back of the brain below the cerebrum and controls the equilibrium and coordination. The brain stem controls involuntary functions, such as respirations, heart rate, temperature control, and nerve transmission. The brain stem is continuous with the **spinal cord**, which is also protected by the meninges and the vertebrae (cervical, thoracic, and lumbar). Cerebrospinal fluid circulates within the subarachnoid space of the brain and the spinal cord.

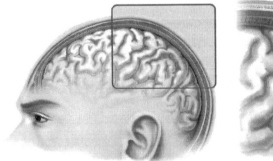 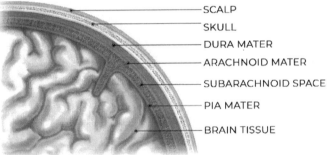

SCALP
SKULL
DURA MATER
ARACHNOID MATER
SUBARACHNOID SPACE
PIA MATER
BRAIN TISSUE

BRAIN AND CERVICAL SPINE INJURIES

Direct injury to **brain** tissue or damage from bleeding inside of the skull may occur with head injury. Altered mental status is likely. Cerebrospinal fluid may leak from the nose/ears. Symptoms include the pupils being unequal, nausea, vomiting, bradycardia (slow heart rate), elevated BP, and irregular breathing.

Prehospital Interventions: Immobilize spine, manage the patient's airway, ventilation, and oxygen supplementation, provide shock prevention, control bleeding, and provide rapid transport.

Suspect injury to the **spine** with motor vehicle/pedestrian accidents, falls, hanging, blunt or penetrating trauma to the head, neck, or torso, diving accidents, and unresponsive trauma patients. Patients may have tenderness in the area, pain on moving, numbness, tingling, or weakness, inability to feel or move below the injury, difficulty breathing, and incontinence (bowel or bladder).

Prehospital Interventions: If patient is responsive, manually stabilize the head and neck in the position found until a cervical collar and backboard are in place. Evaluate the patient's pain, sensations, and ability to move. If patient is unresponsive, stabilize the head and neck as above, manage the airway, ventilation, and oxygenation, question witnesses, and provide rapid transport.

BRAIN INJURIES, THE COUP/CONTRECOUP PATTERN, AND POSTURING

Primary brain injuries are those that result from the original trauma and include direct damage to brain tissue, such as may occur with a gunshot wound. **Secondary brain injuries** result from the effects of the primary injury, such as increasing intracranial pressure, ischemia (most common), hemorrhage, edema, and brain herniation.

Coup/Contrecoup injuries are common in motor vehicle accidents and shaken baby syndrome. With acceleration/deceleration and contact injuries where the head hits a fixed object (such as a windshield) and snaps back from the impact, coup (on the side of impact) and contrecoup (on the opposite side) contusions may both occur.

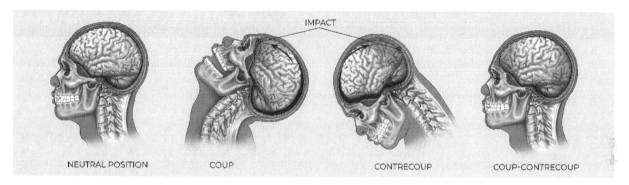

Decerebrate (extension) posturing (with the body stiff, legs straight, feet extended, arms straight, and the head/neck arched back) is associated with severe midbrain damage. **Decorticate (flexion) posturing** (with the body stiff, legs straight, and hands clenched on the chest) is associated with damage to the pathway connecting the brain and spinal cord and may include damage to the cerebral cortex, white matter, or basal ganglia.

DECEREBRATE POSTURING

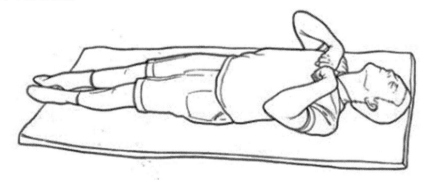

DECORTICATE POSTURING

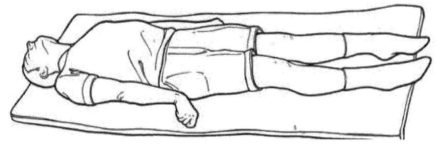

SKULL FRACTURES

The skull is divided into eight cranial bones: one frontal bone (over the frontal lobe), two parietal bones (over the parietal lobes), two temporal bones (over the temporal lobes), one occipital bone (over the occipital lobe and cerebellum), one sphenoid bone (it forms part of the eye orbit), and one ethmoid bone (it separates the nasal cavity from the brain). **Skull fractures** include the following:

- **Basilar**: Occurs in the bones at the base of the brain and can cause severe brain stem damage.
- **Comminuted**: The skull fractures into small pieces.
- **Compound**: A surface laceration extends to a skull fracture, which may be overlooked because of heavy bleeding.
- **Depressed**: May be open and is often comminuted. Pieces of the skull are depressed inward on the brain tissue, often producing dural tears and underlying brain trauma.
- **Linear/hairline**: A skull fracture forms a thin line without any splintering, usually without underlying injury.
- **Diastatic**: Affects children younger than 3 years old, widening the skull sutures.

SKULL BONES AND SUTURES

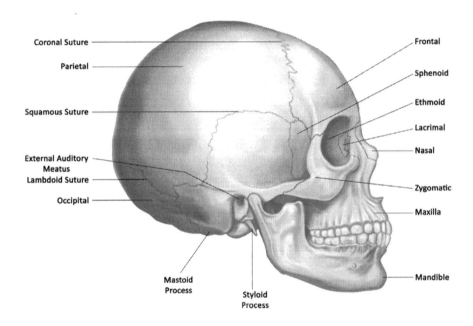

HEAD, SCALP, AND FACIAL INJURIES

Injury	Characteristics	Prehospital
Head	Open: Bleeding. Closed: Swelling and bruising, may have depression of the skull and underlying injury. Battle's sign (bruising over the mastoid process) and/or raccoon eyes (bruising about eyes) may indicate a basal skull fracture.	Apply direct pressure to control the bleeding; apply dry, sterile dressings. Monitor the patient's mental status. Be alert for signs of skull fracture.
Scalp	Copious bleeding may occur. May cause shock in infants and young children. Injuries above the ears increase the risk of brain injury.	As above. Manage the patient's airway, ventilation, and oxygen supplementation if needed. Rapid transport is required with shock. Avoid closing the patient's mouth with bandages.
Facial	May include soft-tissue damage, facial bone fractures (nasal, orbital), eye injuries, and oral/dental injuries (tooth avulsions, mandibular/ maxillary fractures). May have severe swelling, airway compromise, impaired vision, and bloody nose.	Maintain a patent airway, but avoid nasopharyngeal airways; suction as needed; take broken teeth to the hospital; examine the eyes; and control bleeding. Patch both eyes if one or both eyes are injured. Stabilize impaled objects in the eye(s), but remove impaled objects from the cheeks if any bleeding obstructs the patient's airway.

NON-SPINAL NECK INJURIES AND NASAL FRACTURES

Non-spinal neck injuries may result from blunt trauma or penetrating trauma, and they must be carefully assessed for underlying spinal cord injury. Open wounds may bleed profusely, especially if the carotid artery is breached, resulting in rapid exsanguination and death. The airway may be compromised. Difficulty swallowing indicates esophageal injury, whereas voice changes indicate laryngeal injury. Crackling on palpation indicates air in the tissues.

Prehospital Interventions: Apply single-digit (gloved) pressure to control bleeding of the carotid artery or jugular veins; apply an occlusive dressing for an injury to the large vessels after the bleeding is controlled to prevent air from entering the bloodstream, which is life-threatening; and manage the patient's airway/ventilation/oxygen supplementation (advanced life support may be needed). Rapid or air medical transport may be needed.

Nasal fractures (40% of facial fractures) may cause persistent bleeding and should be assessed for drainage of the cerebrospinal fluid and injury of the surrounding structures, including brain injury, skull fracture, and neck and cervical spine injury.

Prehospital Interventions: Control any bleeding, elevate the patient's head, and manage the airway, but do not use a nasopharyngeal airway.

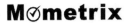

MANDIBULAR FRACTURES, LARYNGOTRACHEAL INJURIES, AND NON-CNS-ASSOCIATED SPINAL TRAUMA

Additional non-CNS fractures of the face, neck and spine include:

- **Mandibular fractures** are most common in males 21 to 30 and result from a blow to the jaw from an assault, motor vehicle accident, or gunshot wound and are often associated with other injuries, such as head injury or midface fractures. Symptoms include malocclusion of teeth, pain, point tenderness, and ecchymosis of the floor of the mouth. **Prehospital Interventions**: Manage the patient's airway/ventilation/oxygen supplementation (avoid the nasal airway), use an ice pack to reduce edema, elevate the patient's head, and monitor him or her closely.

- **Laryngotracheal injuries** result from direct trauma and may result in swelling and hemorrhage. Symptoms include swelling, changes in voice, hemoptysis, subcutaneous emphysema (from open wounds), and structural irregularities. The patient must be assessed for associated injuries. **Prehospital Interventions**: Manage the patient's airway/ventilation/oxygen supplementation because airway obstruction is common, elevate the patient's head, and provide supportive care. May require a surgical airway.

- With **non-CNS-associated spinal trauma**, patients complain of pain and point tenderness, but neurological findings are intact. **Prehospital Interventions**: Provide sitting or standing spinal mobilization and supportive care and manage the patient's airway, ventilation, and oxygen supplementation as needed.

DENTAL INJURIES

Dental fractures, most commonly of the maxillary teeth, may occur in association with other oral and facial injuries and may be overlooked unless a careful dental examination is carried out. Fractures may range from chipping of the enamel to fracture of the tooth root.

Dental avulsions are complete displacement of a tooth from its socket. The tooth may be reimplanted if done within 1-2 hours after displacement, although only permanent teeth are reimplanted, not primary teeth, so question the parents of children to determine if an avulsed tooth is permanent.

Prehospital Interventions: Manage the patient's airway, ventilation, and oxygen supplementation as needed, elevate the patient's head, and place the avulsed tooth in NS for transport.

Nervous System Trauma

CONCUSSIONS

A concussion is a brain injury in which structural damage is not apparent but neurological functioning is impaired. Patients may experience a brief loss of consciousness after a head injury and may experience confusion and even bizarre behavior (if the frontal lobe is affected). Other symptoms include severe headache, somnolence, dizziness, lack of coordination, confusion, disorientation, inappropriate emotional response, nausea, and vomiting. Symptoms are usually transient (lasting from minutes to hours), but up to 50% may have recurrent symptoms (such as difficulty concentrating, headaches, and dizziness) for months. The **American Academy of Neurology classifies concussions** as follows:

- **Grade 1**: Transient confusion without loss of consciousness, with symptoms resolving in <15 minutes
- **Grade 2**: Transient confusion without loss of consciousness, with symptoms resolving in >15 minutes
- **Grade 3**: Any loss of consciousness of any duration

Prehospital Interventions: Provide supportive care and reassurance, monitor vital signs and neurological status for signs of increasing intracranial pressure that may indicate more severe injury, and elevate the patient's head.

SIGNS OF INCREASING INTRACRANIAL PRESSURE

Head trauma may result in **increased intracranial pressure** and cerebral edema. Patients often suffer initial hypertension, which increases intracranial pressure and decreases perfusion, and significant swelling, which also interferes with perfusion, causing hypoxia and hypercapnia (increased carbon dioxide), which trigger increased blood flow. This increased volume at a time when injury impairs autoregulation further increases cerebral edema, which, in turn, increases intracranial pressure and results in a further decrease in perfusion with resultant ischemia (impaired circulation). If the pressure continues to rise, the brain may herniate. The mean arterial pressure must remain between 65 and 150 mmHg for the brain to autoregulate intracranial pressure (the normal pressure is 2–12 mmHg). Symptoms include Cushing's triad: wide pulse pressure, bradycardia, and irregular respirations.

Initially: Decreased levels of consciousness, increased BP, and decreased pulse, Cheyne-Stokes (irregular) respirations, and reactive pupils. Middle brain stem involvement: Wide pulse pressure, bradycardia, pupils sluggish or nonreactive, and hyperventilation. Lower brain stem: Pupil blown on the side of injury, irregular respirations, flaccid response to painful stimulation, and the BP and pulse decrease.

Prehospital Interventions: Elevate the patient's head, manage the patient's airway/ventilation/oxygen supplementation, provide rapid transport, and start an IV access line.

INTRACRANIAL HEMATOMAS

Type	Characteristics	Prehospital
Epidural	Bleeding between the dura and the skull, pushing the brain downward and inward. The hemorrhage is usually caused by arterial tears, so bleeding is often rapid, leading to severe neurological deficits and respiratory arrest. The patient may be lucid and without symptoms for 2–6 hours after the injury.	Provide supportive care, keep the patient's head elevated to reduce intracranial pressure, note neurological status (movement, strength, mental status, pupils equal and reactive or unequal/fixed), and provide rapid transport. Provide an IV access line and fluids.
Subdural	Bleeding between the dura and the arachnoid mater, usually from tears in the cortical veins of the subdural space. It tends to develop more slowly than an epidural hemorrhage. If the bleeding is acute and develops within minutes or hours of injury, then the prognosis is poor. Subacute hematomas that develop more slowly cause varying degrees of injury.	
Intracerebral	Bleeding into the substance of the brain from an artery. Sudden onset; it results in a hemorrhagic stroke with a lack of nutrients and oxygen to parts of the brain. May result from degenerative changes, hypertension, brain tumors, medications, or illicit drugs (crack, cocaine). Symptoms vary depending on the site, but they may include one-sided weakness, paralysis, difficulty speaking, severe headache, and altered mental status.	Provide supportive care, keep the patient's head elevated to reduce intracranial pressure, note neurological status (movement, strength, mental status, pupils equal and reactive or unequal/fixed), provide rapid transport, start an IV access line, and give fluids.
Subarachnoid	Bleeding in the space between the meninges and brain and into the cerebrospinal fluid, usually resulting from aneurysm, arteriovenous malformation (AVM), or trauma. This type of hemorrhage compresses the brain tissue. The first presenting symptoms are severe headache, nausea and vomiting, nuchal rigidity, palsy related to cranial nerve compression, retinal hemorrhages, and papilledema.	

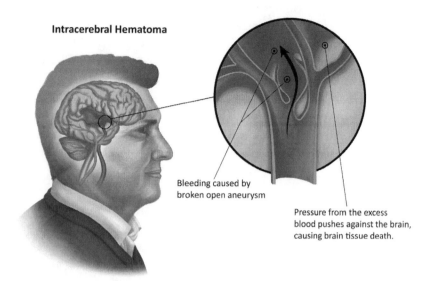

Intracerebral Hematoma

Bleeding caused by broken open aneurysm

Pressure from the excess blood pushes against the brain, causing brain tissue death.

SPINAL INJURIES AND SPINAL CORD INJURIES (SCIs)

Spinal injuries of the vertebrae include fractures, dislocations, open wounds, and flexion and extension injuries. Because the spinal cord lies within the vertebral column, injury to the vertebrae may cause **spinal cord injuries (SCIs)** and disrupt transmissions in nerves that connect the body and the brain. SCI may affect only a few nerves, or they may completely transect the spinal cord, resulting in permanent paralysis below the site of injury. SCIs should be suspected with head trauma, penetrating trauma, direct blunt trauma, falls, diving injuries, motor vehicle accidents, rapid deceleration accidents, and multisystem trauma. Assessment includes evaluating extremity movement, respiration control, sensation, reflexes, pain/tenderness, and vital signs.

Prehospital Interventions: Logroll the patient to examine his or her back, immobilize the patient (seated or standing), apply a rigid cervical collar, lift and move him or her with care, and provide rapid transport. Elevate the torso of children 2–3 cm with padding so that the head is in a neutral position if using an adult immobilization device. Immobilize infants in their car seats, padding all the voids.

Spinal cord injuries (SCIs) may result from blunt trauma (such as automobile accidents), falls from a height, sports injuries, and penetrating trauma (such as a gunshot or knife wound). Damage results from mechanical injury and secondary responses resulting from hemorrhage, edema, and ischemia. The types of symptoms relate to the area and degree of injury, as below:

- **Anterior cord**: This results from pressure/damage to the anterior spinal cord. The posterior column functions remain, so there are sensations of touch, vibration, and position remaining below the injury but with complete paralysis and loss of the sensations of pain and temperature. The prognosis is poor.
- **Brown-Séquard**: The cord is hemisected from penetrating trauma, resulting in spastic paresis, loss of sense of position and vibration on the injured side, and loss of pain and temperature sensation on the other side. The prognosis is good.
- **Posterior cord**: Motor function is preserved but without sensation.
- **Conus medullaris**: Injury to the lower spine (lower lumbar and sacral nerves).

- **Central cord**: This results from hyperextension or hyperflexion and ischemia or stenosis of the cervical spine, causing spinal contusion and quadriparesis (more severe in the upper extremities) with some loss of sensations of pain and temperature. Prognosis is good, but fine motor skills are often impaired in the upper extremities with paresis being more acute distally than proximally in the arms.

Trauma in Special Populations

PREGNANCY AND PEDIATRIC TRAUMA

Pregnancy trauma: The mother and fetus are each considered to be patients. Pregnant patients are susceptible to falls and domestic abuse. Pregnant women have an increased blood volume and heart rate, impaired venous return if in the supine (flat) position in the third trimester, and an increased risk of vomiting and aspiration. Hypovolemia/shock lowers oxygen to the fetus, resulting in fetal stress. Vaginal bleeding may occur.

Prehospital Interventions: Have suction available, monitor the patient's airway, ventilation, and oxygen supplementation with 100% oxygen per nonrebreather mask and ventilation assistance if needed, transport on the left side (tilt the immobilization board if necessary), provide an IV access line and fluids if indicated and rapid transport.

Pediatric trauma: Assess the pediatric triangle (appearance, work of breathing, and circulation). The respiration rate varies with age, but the use of accessory muscles and sternal retraction indicate respiratory distress. Assess the brachial pulse in infants—a slow pulse indicates hypoxia.

Prehospital Interventions: Manage hypovolemia/shock, prevent hypothermia, and manage the patient's airway, ventilation, and oxygen supplementation as needed. Ventilate if he or she is bradycardic (BVM is preferred for children).

TRAUMA IN GERIATRIC PATIENTS

Geriatric patients are more susceptible to trauma because of aging processes, and they may be less able to maintain normal vital signs during hemorrhage. Polypharmacy is common, and medications may affect vital signs and blood clotting. The risk of cerebral bleeding is increased because of brain shrinkage. The cough reflex may be lessened. Fractures are common because of osteoporosis, especially hip fractures.

Prehospital Interventions: Splint fractures, monitor the patient's airway, ventilation, and oxygen supplementation, monitor oxygenation with pulse oximetry, suction if necessary, and check the mouth for dentures (which may obstruct the airway). Spinal curvature may require padding of the spinal board.

TRAUMA IN THE COGNITIVELY IMPAIRED PATIENT

Disorders that result in cognitive impairment may include Alzheimer's or other forms of dementia, traumatic brain injuries, strokes, Down syndrome, and autistic spectrum disorders. Patients may be more at risk of trauma, and assessment and history taking may be difficult. Perceptions of pain may be altered, and psychological reactions may vary.

Prehospital Interventions: Remain supportive, reassure the patient, obtain information from the caregiver if necessary, and treat as indicated by the patient's condition.

Environmental Emergencies

TEMPERATURE-RELATED TRAUMA

GENERALIZED HYPOTHERMIA

Generalized hypothermia occurs when the body temperature falls to below-normal levels:

- Mild: 34–36 °C (93.2–96.8 °F)
- Moderate: 30–34 °C (86.0–93.2 °F)
- Severe: <30 °C (<86.0 °F)

Contributing factors include wet and cold environments, wind, age (geriatric/pediatric), medical conditions, substance abuse (alcohol, drugs), and poison. Up to 50% of trauma patients with severe injuries become hypothermic because of exposure, blood loss, shock, and standard procedures (such as administration of cold fluids and clothing removal). Indications of hypothermia include cold skin, shivering, decreased mental status (confusion, memory loss, lethargy, dizziness, mood changes, impaired judgment, difficulty speaking), decreased sensation of touch, decreased motor function (muscle rigidity, stiff posture, muscle/joint stiffness), and bradycardia.

Prehospital Interventions: Remove the patient from the cold environment, remove any wet clothing, wrap in warm blankets, begin CPR if no pulse is obtained after 30–45 seconds of assessment, and use an AED if it indicates the need to defibrillate.

FROSTBITE/FREEZING

Frostbite is tissue damage from freezing, most often affecting the nose, ears, and distal extremities (hands/feet). The affected part feels numb and aches or throbs, becoming hard and insensate as the tissue freezes, resulting in circulatory impairment, necrosis of tissue, and gangrene. **Degrees of frostbite/freezing** are as follows:

1. Partial freezing with erythema and mild edema, stinging, burning, and throbbing pain.
2. Full-thickness freezing with increased edema in 3–4 hours and clear blisters in 6–24 hours; sloughing of skin with eschar formation, numbness, and then aching and throbbing pain.
3. Full-thickness freezing into the subdermal tissue with cyanosis, hemorrhagic blisters, skin necrosis, a "wooden" feeling, severe burning, throbbing, and shooting pains.
4. Freezing extends into the subcutaneous tissue (muscles, tendons, and bones) with a mottled appearance, non-blanching cyanosis, and eventually deep black eschar.

Prehospital Interventions: Remove the patient from the cold environment with care, remove wet clothing, cover the patient with a blanket, remove jewelry, manually stabilize the affected area, and transport rapidly. Do NOT break blisters, rub or massage the area, apply heat, rewarm if the area may refreeze, allow the patient to walk, or give him or her anything by mouth.

HEAT-RELATED ILLNESSES

Heat-related illnesses include:

- **Heat Stress**: Increased temperature causes dehydration. Symptoms may include swelling of the hands and feet, flushing, itching, sunburn, dizziness, muscle cramps, and hyperventilation. The patient's temperature is normal.
  Prehospital Interventions: Remove the patient from heat, give fluids to rehydrate, and give oxygen with a nonrebreather mask.
- **Heat Exhaustion**: Dehydration results in sodium depletion. Symptoms may include flu-like symptoms, headache, dizziness, fainting, nausea, vomiting, weakness, muscle cramping, rapid pulse, diaphoresis, and cold clammy skin. The patient's temperature is usually <41 °C (105.8 °F), and it may be normal.
  Prehospital Interventions: Remove the patient from heat; use evaporative cooling techniques such as ice packs to the axilla, groin, and neck; rehydrate (half glass of water every 15-20 minutes). Give oxygen as above.
- **Heat Stroke**: There are two types, which may progress to multiorgan dysfunction syndrome with liver and kidney failure, and death. **Exertional**: Sudden onset after exertion. The patient's temperature varies because he or she is still sweating; there is diaphoresis, syncope, and loss of consciousness. **Non-exertional**: Sudden onset after heat exposure. The temperature is usually >41 °C (105.8 °F) rectally or >39.4 °C (102.9 °F) orally. There can be mild irritability, decorticate posturing, seizures, coma, and tachycardia.
  Prehospital Interventions: Remove the patient from heat, apply evaporative cooling and ice packs as above; provide airway/ventilation/oxygenation support as needed, IV access line and fluids, and rapid transport.

SUBMERSION/DROWNING

Submersion may cause aspiration (wet drowning) or trigger severe laryngospasm (dry drowning), although some people will be pulled from the water still breathing. **Drowning** is the leading cause of death in children younger than age 5, and it is the second leading cause of death in children younger than age 15. Most infant submersions are in bathtubs and result from intentional injury or lack of supervision. Adolescent and adult submersions are often related to drugs, alcohol, or risk-taking behaviors. Submersion asphyxiation can cause profound damage to multiple organ systems, including the brain, heart, and lungs, from a lack of oxygen and aspiration. Hypothermia related to near drowning has some protective effect because blood is shunted to the brain and heart. Indications of submersion include coughing, vomiting, difficulty breathing, and respiratory and cardiac arrest.

Prehospital Interventions: Initiate CPR if the patient is in arrest, manage the patient's airway/ventilation/oxygen supplementation with 100% oxygen (may need intubation), place him or her in the recovery position if he or she is unconscious or vomiting, provide suction as needed, start an IV access line, and provide rapid transport.

Multisystem Trauma

MULTI-SYSTEM TRAUMA

Multi-system trauma involves injury to more than one major system, which is quite common. Care includes the following points:

- Ensure the safety of the patient and all rescue personnel and determine the need for additional resources.
- Consider the mechanism of injury and identify and manage life-threatening conditions.
- Manage the patient's airway, ventilation, and oxygen supplementation (high concentration) as well as necessary spinal immobilization with him or her in a lying/sitting position, and make positioning decisions.
- Control hemorrhage, provide shock therapy, and maintain body temperature.
- Splint musculoskeletal injuries.
- Suspect additional injuries.
- Prioritize interventions and continue care en route rather than delaying transport.
- Evaluate the patient's condition by the injuries sustained (bleeding, difficulty breathing, lack of pulse) rather than by the patient's response (screaming, yelling).
- Complete the primary and secondary assessments, and obtain a medical history.
- Platinum ten—the first 10 minutes on the scene in which the patient should be extricated and stabilization efforts should be started.
- Golden hour—the first 60 minutes during which the patient should be stabilized and transported to the receiving facility.
- Notify the receiving facility so that resources are prepared.

BLAST INJURIES

Blast injuries may result from high-order explosives (TNT, nitroglycerin) or low-order explosives (pipe bombs, Molotov cocktails). Enclosed explosions usually cause more injury than do open-air blasts. Blast waves occur only with high-order explosives and result from high-pressure impulses. Blast wind may occur with either type of explosive and involves superheated air. Ground shock may cause further injury. Immediate death may occur.

Injuries may include the following:

- **Primary**: Blast wave injury affects gas-filled organs/structures including the lungs, eardrum, abdomen, eyes, and brain (20% of victims).
- **Secondary**: Penetrating injuries from flying shrapnel affecting any part of the body along with abrasions, contusions, and lacerations. (Secondary injury is the most common cause of death.)
- **Tertiary**: Injuries from being thrown by blast wind, such as fractures, spinal and brain injuries, and traumatic amputations.
- **Quaternary**: Other injuries and complications, such as difficulty breathing because of smoke inhalation, burns, and crush injuries.

Prehospital Interventions:

- Be alert for a second explosive device or a device on a victim (who may be a perpetrator).
- Carry out rapid triage.
- Control any bleeding and manage shock.
- Manage the patient's airway, ventilation, and oxygen supplementation. Provide CPR if necessary.
- Splint musculoskeletal injuries.
- Start an IV access and give fluid resuscitation.
- Provide rapid transport.

Medical/Obstetrics/Gynecology

Neurological Emergencies

NEUROLOGICAL SYSTEM

The neurological (nervous) system consists of the **central nervous system (CNS)**, which contains the brain, spinal cord and nerves, and the **peripheral nervous system (PNS)**, which contains the sensory neurons, ganglia (nerve clusters), and nerves connecting to the CNS. The brain consists of the **cerebrum** (frontal, temporal, parietal, and occipital lobes); the **cerebellum**; and the **brain stem**, which is continuous with the spinal cord. The PNS is divided into the **autonomic nervous system (ANS)** and the **somatic nervous system (SoNS)**. The autonomic nervous system controls the body's organs and maintains homeostasis (balance). Functions of the ANS include control of the heart rate and function, respiration, digestion, sexual arousal, and other systems. The SoNS comprises cranial and spinal nerves that connect the CNS to the skeletal muscles and skin. The SoNS is the voluntarily controlled component of the PNS, and it receives and responds to external sensory stimuli from the skin and sensory organs.

> **Review Video: Brain Anatomy**
> Visit mometrix.com/academy and enter code: 222476

GLASGOW COMA SCALE (GCS)

The Glasgow coma scale (GCS) measures the depth and duration of coma or impaired level of consciousness; it is a critical part of the neurological assessment and, when trended, can mark progress/recovery or neurological decline. The GCS measures three parameters: best eye response, best verbal response, and best motor response, with a total possible score that ranges from 3 to 15. The same scale is used with slight modifications for infants.

Eye opening	4: Spontaneous 3: To verbal stimuli 2: To pain (not of face) 1: No response
Verbal	5: Oriented 4: Conversation confused, but can answer questions 3: Uses inappropriate words 2: Speech incomprehensible 1: No response
Motor	6: Moves on command 5: Moves purposefully respond pain 4: Withdraws in response to pain 3: Decorticate posturing (flexion) in response to pain 2: Decerebrate posturing (extension) in response to pain 1: No response

Injuries/conditions are classified according to the total score: 3-8 Coma; ≤8 Severe head injury likely requiring intubation; 9-12 Moderate head injury; 13-15 Mild head injury.

> **Review Video: Glasgow Coma Scale**
> Visit mometrix.com/academy and enter code: 133399

94

STROKES

Strokes result from interruption of blood flow to an area of the brain.

- **Ischemic strokes** (80%) are caused by blockage of an artery supplying the brain, usually from a thrombus (blood clot) or embolus (traveling clot).
- **Hemorrhagic strokes** (20%) result from a ruptured cerebral artery, causing not only a lack of oxygen and nutrients but also edema (swelling) that causes widespread pressure and damage. With both types, patients may experience weakness, paralysis, and loss of sensation in one or more extremities; difficulty speaking or loss of speech; vision impairment; difficulty swallowing; headache; an altered state of consciousness (confusion, disorientation); or coma.
- **Transient ischemic attacks** (TIAs) from small clots cause similar but short-lived (minutes to hours) symptoms. Emergent treatment includes placing the patient in the semi-Fowlers or Fowler's position and administering oxygen. The patient may require oral suctioning if the secretions pool. The patient's airway, breathing, and circulation should be assessed. Patients should be transported immediately to the receiving facility because thrombolytic therapy to dissolve blood clots should be administered within 1-3 hours.

> **Review Video: Overview of Strokes**
> Visit mometrix.com/academy and enter code: 310572

CINCINNATI PREHOSPITAL STROKE SCALE

The Cincinnati Prehospital Stroke Scale should be administered to any patient who is suspected of having a stroke. The patient may be experiencing a stroke if he tests positive for any of the three signs and should be transported to the receiving facility as soon as possible.

Signs	Directions to patient	Abnormal results
Facial drooping	Smile. Show your teeth.	One side of the face is weak or paralyzed and doesn't move as well as the other.
Arm drifting	Close your eyes and hold your arms out straight and hold them there for 10 seconds.	One arm doesn't move at all or drifts downward.
Speaking abnormality	Repeat after me: "Don't count your chickens before they are hatched."	Patient slurs words, uses inappropriate words, or is unable to respond.

LOS ANGELES PREHOSPITAL STROKE SCREEN

The Los Angeles Prehospital Stroke Screen is used to assess patients in a prehospital setting who have symptoms that suggest a stroke (such as altered state of consciousness, difficulty speaking, one-sided weakness, or paralysis). The results are positive for stroke if all criteria are met or are unable to be measured and the physical exam shows an unequal response. Note: A patient may still be having a stroke even if all the criteria are not met.

General criteria	Yes	No	Unknown
Age >45			
No history of epilepsy or seizures			
Onset of symptoms <24 hours			
Patient was able to walk before the onset of symptoms			
Blood glucose between 60 and 400 mg/dL			

Physical criteria	Equal	Right	Left
Facial smile	Normal	Droop	Droop
Grip strength	Normal	Weak or no grip	Weak or no grip
Arm strength	Normal	Drifts or falls down	Drifts or falls down

SEIZURES

GRAND MAL SEIZURES

Seizures are sudden, involuntary, abnormal electrical disturbances in the brain that can manifest as alterations of consciousness, spastic tonic and clonic movements, convulsions, and loss of consciousness.

- **Tonic-clonic (grand mal)**: Occurs without warning.
  - *Tonic period* (10–30 seconds): The eyes roll upward with loss of consciousness, the arms flex, and the body stiffens in symmetric contractions with cyanosis and salivating.
  - *Clonic period* (usually 30 seconds or longer): Violent rhythmic jerking with contraction and relaxation and sometimes incontinence of urine and feces.

During the seizure, the patient's head and body should be protected from injury but no attempt should be made to insert anything into the mouth or restrain the patient. If possible, the patient should be screened from spectators and turned onto his or her side (the recovery position) to prevent aspiration. Following seizures, there may be confusion, disorientation, and impairment of motor activity and speech and vision for several hours. Headache, nausea, and vomiting may occur.

> **Review Video: Seizures**
> Visit mometrix.com/academy and enter code: 977061

Prehospital Interventions: Monitor the airway, breathing, and circulation and suction. Administer oxygen as needed. Insert a nasopharyngeal airway for assisted ventilation if the patient is cyanotic.

PARTIAL SEIZURES

Partial seizures are caused by an electrical discharge to a localized area of the cerebral cortex, such as the frontal, temporal, or parietal lobes with seizure characteristics related to the area of involvement. They may begin in a focal area and become generalized, often preceded by an aura.

- **Simple partial**: Unilateral motor symptoms including somatosensory, psychic, and autonomic.
  - *Aversive*: Eyes and head are turned away from the focal side.
  - *Sylvan* (usually during sleep): Tonic-clonic movements of the face, salivation, and arrested speech.
- **Special sensory**: Various sensations (numbness, tingling, prickling, or pain) spreading from one area. May include visual sensations, posturing, or hypertonia. These are rare in patients <8 years old.
- **Complex (psychomotor)**: There is no loss of consciousness, but there may be altered levels of consciousness, and patients may be nonresponsive with amnesia. May involve complex sensorium with bad tastes, auditory or visual hallucinations, and a feeling of déjà vu or strong fear. Patients may carry out repetitive activities, such as walking, running, smacking lips, chewing, or drawling. Patients are rarely aggressive. The seizure is usually followed by prolonged drowsiness and confusion. Occurs from age 3 through adolescence.

NEUROLOGICAL ASSESSMENT
ASSESSING THE PATIENT'S LEVEL OF CONSCIOUSNESS

The **AVPU** is a quick assessment done to determine the **patient's level of consciousness**. This may be one of the first assessments done when initially attending to a patient.

Alert, voice, pain, unresponsive (AVPU)		
A Alert and awake; aware of person, place, time, and condition. Follows commands. Pediatric: Active and responds to external stimuli and to caregiver.	Yes	No
V Responds to verbal stimuli, but the eyes do not open spontaneously. Pediatric: Responds only when the caregiver calls the child's name.	Yes	No
P Responds to painful stimuli, such as pinching the skin/earlobe, but not to verbal stimuli. Pediatric: Responds only to painful stimuli, such as pinching the nailbed.	Yes	No
U Unresponsive; does not respond to painful or verbal stimuli. Pediatric: Unresponsive.	Yes	No

ASSESSMENT OF A PATIENT'S MENTAL STATUS

When assessing a patient's mental status, make note of the following:

- **Level of consciousness**: Using the AVPU assessment.
- **Posture and behavior**: Abnormal findings include restlessness, agitation, bizarre posturing, catatonia (immobility), and tics or other abnormal movements.
- **Dress, grooming, and hygiene**: Kempt or unkempt, clean or dirty.
- **Facial expressions**: May vary widely (anxious, depressed, angry, sad, elated, or fearful). Note whether the patient's expressions seem appropriate to the situation/words.
- **Speech/Language**: Quantity, rate, fluency, appropriate/inappropriate. Note aphasia (inability to speak and/or understand words), dysphonia (abnormal voice/difficulty speaking), or dysarthria (difficulty speaking words).
- **Mood**: Nature and duration of the patient's current mood. Note suicidal ideation.
- **Thoughts/Perceptions**: Note logic, relevance, and organization of thoughts and abnormal findings, such as thought blocking (sudden period of silence in the middle of a sentence while speaking), flight of ideas (racing thoughts), incoherence, confabulation (producing distorted memories), loose association (responses not connected to questions or one sentence not connected to the next), or transference (redirecting emotions to a substitute). Note homicidal or suicidal thoughts, obsessions, compulsions, delusions, illusions, and hallucinations.
- **Judgment**: Note the patient's insight, ability to make decisions, and ability to plan.

CAUSES OF ALTERED MENTAL STATUS

Altered mental status occurs because brain functioning is disrupted. Signs of altered mental status may be subtle (such as slight agitation, lethargy, sleepiness, or forgetfulness) or more obvious (such as disorientation, confusion, personality changes, violent behavior, somnolence, seizures, and coma). An **altered mental status** may occur abruptly or may have a slower onset, depending on the cause:

- **Inadequate oxygenation**: Brain cells can only survive about 6 minutes without oxygen, but damage begins to occur after about 60 seconds.
- **Inadequate ventilation**: Even if oxygen is plentiful, gas exchange is inadequate with impaired ventilation.
- **Overdose of medication**: May occur with numerous drugs, including opioids/narcotics (such as heroin and oxycodone), antipsychotics, hallucinogens, inhalants, cocaine, methamphetamines, and benzodiazepines.
- **Poisoning**: Includes arsenic; lead; cyanide; and overdose of medications such as acetaminophen, clonidine, salicylates, calcium channel blockers, and beta blockers.
- **Infection**: Systemic infections (sepsis), brain abscesses, chronic infections (human immunodeficiency virus/acquired immune deficiency syndrome [HIV/AIDS]).
- **Psychological/psychiatric condition**: Includes bipolar disorder, schizophrenia, post-traumatic stress disorder (PTSD), and depression.
- **Diabetes**: Hyperglycemia and hypoglycemia (especially insulin reaction).

AEIOU TIPS MNEMONIC TO OUTLINE THE POTENTIAL CAUSES FOR ALTERED MENTAL STATUS

Many different conditions can lead to altered mental status, and the EMS provider should consider all possibilities because emergent treatment may vary depending on the cause. Always check for medical alert jewelry. The following **AEIOU TIPS mnemonic** is a helpful guide to recalling potential causes:

A	Alcohol/Acidosis	Note the smell of alcohol, empty alcohol containers.
E	Endocrine/Epilepsy	Consider electrolyte imbalance, encephalopathy; note oral trauma, urinary incontinence.
I	Infection	Consider urinary infection in older adults, meningitis, encephalitis, sepsis.
O	Opiates/ Overdose	Note if the pupils are constricted, drug paraphernalia, history of drug taking, empty medicine containers.
U	Uremia/ Underdose	Note generalized edema, history of kidney failure, failure to take prescribed medicines.
T	Trauma	Consider head injury, excessive bleeding, assault.
I	Insulin	Check refrigerator/medicine cabinet for diabetes medications; check the blood glucose level.
P	Poisoning/Psychosis	Note any history of psychiatric illness; observe the environment for poisons.
S	Stroke/Seizures	Note one-sided weakness, incontinence, difficulty speaking, somnolence.

MENTAL STATUS EXAM (MSE)

Mental status is usually assessed through normal interactions, and the **mental status exam** (MSE) can be used as a guide when assessing patients. Some components require only observation, whereas others require questioning. Components include the following:

- **Appearance**: Kempt, unkempt
- **Behavior/attitude**: Appropriate, inappropriate
- **Consciousness/alertness**: Conscious, arousable, able to focus
- **Orientation**: Person, place, time, event
- **Speech/language**: Normal, abnormal, bizarre, tone, volume
- **Thought processes/content**: Logical/Illogical thinking, delusions, hallucinations, paranoia, fixations, suicidal ideation
- **Affect**: Flat (no expression), blunted (little expression), broad (a wide range of expressions), inappropriate (inconsistent), and restricted (one expression at all times)
- **Mood**: Happy, sad, depressed, elated, withdrawn
- **Attention span**: Appropriate, short, scattered
- **Memory**: Intact, short- or long-term memory loss
- **Judgment/reasoning**: Ability to make reasonable decisions and ability to understand and reason
- **Suicidal or homicidal ideation**: Present, absent

ASSESSMENT OF MEMORY AND ATTENTION

Techniques for the assessment of memory and attention include the following:

- **Orientation**: Ask patient questions to determine if he or she knows person (their name), place (where they are), time (date and hour), and event (what's happening). If a patient knows all of that information, then he or she is oriented ×4.
- **Digit span test**: Tell or show the patient a sequence of six or seven numbers and ask him or her to recall and repeat them.
- **Word recall**: Name three unrelated items and ask the patient to remember them. Wait a few minutes, and then ask the patient to name the items.
- **Serial 7s test**: Ask the patient to count backward from 100 by 7s (100, 93, 86. . .).
- **Spell backward test**: Ask the patient to spell "world" backward (D-L-R-O-W).
- **Remote memory**: Ask the patient to tell her birthdate or that of a close family member.
- **Recent memory**: Ask the patient to describe events earlier in the day.
- **Current memory**: Ask the patient to recall your name or the name of someone else present and to whom the patient was recently introduced.

HEADACHES AND MIGRAINES

Types of headaches/migraines include the following:

- **Tension**: Steady, constant pressure-like pain usually starting in the forehead, temples, or the back of the neck.
- **Cluster**: Unilateral, occurring one to eight times daily, often for several weeks and associated with severe pain in the eye and orbit and radiating to the face and temporal area.
- **Migraine**: Severe recurring headaches often characterized by a prodrome phase, aura phase, headache phase, and recovery phase.
- **Head/neck trauma-related headaches**: Vary but may start at neck or shoulders and radiate to the top of the head.
- **Bleeding/stroke-related headaches**:
  - *Epidural*: Sudden severe, intense
  - *Subdural*: Progressive headache worsening over time
  - *Subarachnoid*: "Thunderclap" severe headache with abrupt onset; may be worse at the back of the head
  - *Stroke*: Tension-type headache with the site of pain relating to the area of injury, often associated with alterations in mental status and other symptoms, such as weakness, paralysis, nausea and vomiting, and photophobia.

STATUS EPILEPTICUS

Status epilepticus (SE) is usually generalized tonic-clonic seizures that are characterized by a series of seizures with the intervening time being too short for the regaining of consciousness. The constant seizures and periods of apnea can lead to exhaustion, respiratory failure with hypoxemia and hypercapnia, hyperthermia, cardiac failure, and death. SE may result from uncontrolled epilepsy, noncompliance with anticonvulsive treatment, stroke, encephalopathy, drug toxicity, brain trauma, brain tumors (neoplasms), and metabolic disorders. SE is life threatening, so treatment should begin as soon as possible.

Prehospital Interventions:

- Place an intravenous (IV) line.
- If opioid drug intoxication is the suspected cause, administer naloxone.
- Administer midazolam (intramuscular [IM]) (5 to 10 mg), lorazepam (IV), or diazepam (IV) to control seizures.
- Intubate and ventilate if in respiratory distress.
- Provide supportive care for seizures to prevent injury.
- Control hyperthermia with room-temperature water to skin and an IV normal saline (NS) bolus of 500 mL.

Gastrointestinal Emergencies

Gastrointestinal (GI) Tract

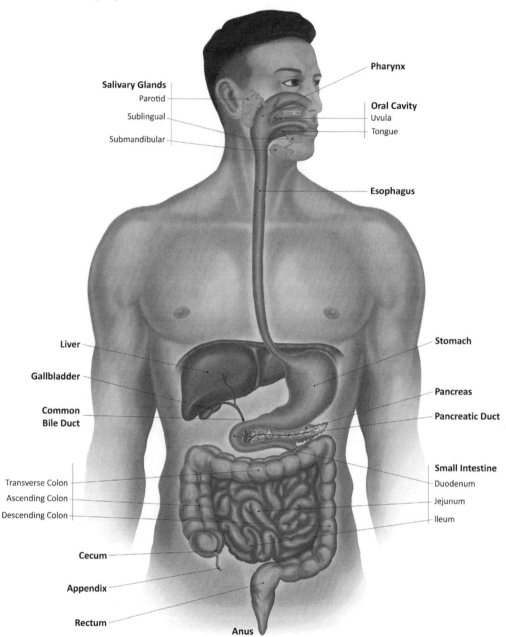

Pharynx

Salivary Glands
Parotid
Sublingual
Submandibular

Oral Cavity
Uvula
Tongue

Esophagus

Liver

Stomach

Gallbladder

Pancreas

Common Bile Duct

Pancreatic Duct

Small Intestine
Duodenum
Jejunum
Ileum

Transverse Colon
Ascending Colon
Descending Colon

Cecum

Appendix

Rectum

Anus

Elements of the **gastrointestinal tract**:

- **Mouth**: Chews, moistens, begins carbohydrate hydrolysis (the breakdown of food by enzymes), creates a bolus of food. Connected to the esophagus by the pharynx.
- **Esophagus**: Transports a bolus through the lower esophageal sphincter (which prevents backflow up the esophagus) to the stomach by peristalsis (wavelike contractions)
- **Stomach**: Churns, secretes acids and enzymes, begins hydrolysis of proteins, and creates chyme (a more fluid substance)
- **Small intestine (about 20 feet long)**:
  - Duodenum: Accepts chyme and digests food to prepare for absorption
  - Jejunum: Absorbs most of the nutrients from the food, including vitamin B_{12}; accepts bile from the liver and gallbladder to digest fats and pancreatic enzymes from the pancreas to digest proteins, fats, and carbohydrates
  - Ileum: Contains the ileocecal valve, which controls the flow of chyme into the large intestine
- **Large intestine (about 5 feet long)**:
  - Cecum: Reabsorbs fluids and electrolytes
  - Appendix: Is believed to store useful gut bacteria
  - Ascending, transverse, descending colon: Reabsorbs water, vitamin K, and electrolytes to form feces
- **Rectum**: Stores feces
- **Anus**: Contains sphincters that control the expelling of feces

> **Review Video: Gastrointestinal System**
> Visit mometrix.com/academy and enter code: 378740

GASTROINTESTINAL BLEEDING

Gastrointestinal bleeding may occur anywhere within the GI system but is most common from the upper GI. Bleeding may range from slow and insidious to massive hemorrhage. Causes include esophageal inflammatory bowel disease (IBD), HIV/CMV infection, polyps, cancer, hemorrhoids, diverticulosis, ulcers, varices (associated with liver disease), Meckel's diverticulum, anticoagulation, and overuse of NSAIDS, such as aspirin and ibuprofen, so history can provide important clues. Output may help to differentiate upper GI bleeding from lower:

- Hematemesis/Coffee ground emesis: Upper GI
- Melena (dark, tarry, foul-smelling stool): Upper GI
- Hematochezia (bright bloody stool)/Clots: Lower GI or massive upper GI
- Bright blood about outside of stool: Hemorrhoids, lower GI

Prehospital Interventions: Assess vital signs and oxygen saturation, abdominal tenderness, and signs of hypovolemic shock (pallor, hypotension, tachycardia, cool/clammy skin, loss of consciousness). With rectal bleeding, place absorbent pads on stretcher. Start two large-bore IVs and begin resuscitation with 1-2 L of crystalloid (NS/Lactated Ringer's) with signs of hypovolemia. Provide supplemental oxygen as needed to maintain oxygen saturation above 94%. Monitor ECG readings. With upper GI bleeding, vomiting, and abdominal distention, insertion of an NG tube may be indicated. Provide blood transfusions if indicated and available.

PERITONITIS

Peritonitis is a bacterial infection of the peritoneum (lining of the abdominal cavity) that can lead to septicemia and death. Patients with kidney failure (especially those patients on peritoneal dialysis), liver disease, or infection of the GI tract are especially at risk. Other causes include an abdominal wound, ruptured appendix, perforated colon, diverticulitis, abdominal surgery, and inflammatory bowel disease. Symptoms include signs of acute abdomen: abdominal pain and distension, rigid abdomen, nausea and vomiting, diarrhea, fever, and chills. Other symptoms may include decreased urine output, excessive thirst, and tachycardia (rapid pulse). Peritonitis may be associated with ulcerative diseases, such as Crohn's disease (open sores through all layers of the walls of any part of the GI tract, most commonly in the ileum) and ulcerative colitis (open sores in the inner lining of the colon).

Prehospital Interventions: Obtain an accurate medical history, note the condition of the abdomen with gentle palpation, provide supplemental oxygen/ventilation as needed, and position the patient for comfort because he or she may be experiencing severe pain.

ULCERATIVE COLITIS AND CROHN'S DISEASE

Ulcerative colitis is superficial inflammation of the mucosa of the colon and rectum, causing ulcerations ranging from pinpoint to extensive. Ulcerations may bleed and produce purulent material. The mucosa of the bowel becomes swollen, erythematous (red), and granular. Onset is usually between ages 15 and 30. Ulcerative colitis may affect only the rectum, the entire colon, or only the left colon. Indications include abdominal pain (usually absent or mild unless disease is severe), bloody diarrhea, rectal bleeding, fecal urgency, and tenesmus (a constant feeling of having to defecate).

> **Review Video: Ulcerative Colitis**
> Visit mometrix.com/academy and enter code: 584881

Crohn's disease is chronic inflammation of any area of the GI system but most commonly the small intestine and the beginning of the large intestine, resulting in ulcers that may involve the full thickness of the intestinal wall. An acute flare-up may mimic appendicitis. Indications include diarrhea (watery), rectal bleeding, abdominal cramping and pain (usually in the right lower quadrant), nausea, vomiting, fever, and night sweats.

Prehospital Interventions: Provide supportive care, manage the patient's airway/ventilation/oxygen supplementation (to maintain oxygen saturation of ≥94%), and provide shock treatment per protocol if necessary.

Immunological Emergencies

ALLERGIC REACTIONS AND ANAPHYLAXIS

Allergic reactions are the response of the body's immune system to an antigen (substance), such as peanuts or shellfish. The body produces antibodies (immunoglobulins, such as IgE or non-IgE) that can identify and attempt to neutralize or destroy antigens. Allergic responses may be mild (local rash, redness, itching, swelling, congestion), moderate (generalized itching, difficulty breathing), or severe (life-threatening anaphylaxis).

With **anaphylaxis**, an antigen triggers the release of substances that affect the skin, cardiopulmonary system, and GI tract. Histamine causes initial redness and swelling by inducing vasodilation. In some cases, initial reactions may be mild, but subsequent contact can cause a severe, life-threatening response. Symptoms include a sudden onset of weakness, dizziness, and confusion; tachycardia; generalized swelling; itching; severe low BP leading to shock; airway obstruction; nausea and vomiting; hives; diarrhea; seizures; coma; and death.

Prehospital Interventions: Inject epinephrine to the lateral thigh and repeat every 5-10 minutes as needed; provide an antihistamine (diphenhydramine) for itching, a vasopressor for hypotension, a bronchodilator (salbutamol/magnesium sulfate) for respiratory distress, supplemental oxygen/ventilation, intubation if necessary, an IV access line, and immediate transport.

> **Review Video: Immune System**
> Visit mometrix.com/academy and enter code: 622899

Infectious Disease

INFECTIOUS AND CONTAGIOUS DISEASES

Infectious diseases, which may be communicable or noncommunicable, are those that are caused when microorganisms (such as bacteria, viruses, retroviruses, protozoa, helminths [worms], and fungi) invade the body and cause disease.

- **Noncommunicable diseases** may spread from an environmental source, such as contaminated water or food (such as with food poisoning), or from insects that carry the disease (such as with Lyme disease). However, they do not spread from person to person, so only standard precautions are needed when caring for these patients.
- **Contagious (communicable) diseases** are infections that are spreadable from person to person. They may be transmitted through direct physical contact and sneezing or coughing as well as through contact with blood or other body fluids (feces, urine, semen, or sweat). With contagious diseases, the type of precautions needed depends on the mode of infection, and they may range from contact to droplet to airborne precautions. The type of PPE needed also varies.

PROCEDURES FOR EXPOSURE/CONTAMINATION

Any exposure/contamination should be reported at hand-off and to the appropriate infection control person following protocols, and follow-up care should be sought if necessary. **Decontamination procedures** are as follows:

- **Skin**: Cleanse the area thoroughly with soap and water.
- **Eyes**: Flush with water for 20 minutes.
- **Needlestick**: Wash the area with soap and water and report immediately.
- **Clothing**: Remove the clothing as soon as possible, and wash visible soiling of skin with soap and water if a shower is not immediately available, but shower as soon as possible. Clothes should be washed separately in a washing machine at the workplace.
- **Equipment/Vehicle**: Clean thoroughly with disinfectant. Dispose of equipment if unable to adequately decontaminate it.

When reporting exposures/contamination, note the type of exposure, the date and time of exposure, circumstances, actions taken to decontaminate, and any other required information.

DECONTAMINATING AN AMBULANCE

Decontaminating an ambulance begins with the removal of any debris with sharps being deposited in a sharps container and soiled linen being red-bagged. Then, the equipment and surfaces that have had contact with a patient or with contaminated materials must be cleaned, disinfected, or sterilized, depending on the type of equipment/surface and the type of contamination. Between patients, surfaces and equipment should be wiped down with a disinfectant, such as a 1:100 chlorine bleach solution or premixed wipes. Alcohol-based products are effective for many organisms, but not for *Clostridium difficile* (which is spread through fecal contamination). If equipment is left with a patient at a receiving facility, that facility must clean the equipment or place it in a red bag before returning it. At the end of the day, the entire ambulance should be cleaned. Various methods of sterilization, including the use of fogging agents and UV lights, are available. All cleaning procedures must be recorded for compliance purposes.

INFECTIOUS VIRAL DISEASES

Disease	Vaccine	Characteristics/Considerations
Chickenpox (varicella)	Varicella or MMRV	Fever, flu-like symptoms, headache, and generalized vesicular rash. Complications: Viral encephalitis, meningitis, pneumonia, Reye's syndrome. Use contact and airborne precautions until lesions are crusted over in 1–3 weeks.
Mumps	MMR or MMRV	Fever, earache, swelling of parotid gland(s), pain, stiff neck (15%). Complications: Spreads to testicles or other parts of the body (heart, kidneys, ovaries, pancreas, brain). There may be hearing impairment. Use standard and droplet precautions.
German measles (rubella)	MMR or MMRV	Low-grade fever, headache, sore throat, anorexia for 1–5 days and then a pink maculopapular rash on the face progressing to the neck, trunk, and legs. Complications: Encephalitis, arthritis (in adolescents). The disease is usually mild, but it poses a risk for the fetus if the mother is infected. Use standard and droplet precautions.
Measles (rubeola)	MMR or MMRV	High fever, conjunctivitis, cough, photophobia, Koplik spots in the mouth, and then a generalized dark-red maculopapular rash, subsiding in 4–7 days. Complications: Diarrhea, otitis media, bronchitis, pneumonia, encephalitis, death. Use airborne precautions while the patient is contagious.
Whooping cough (pertussis)	Dtap or tDap	**Catarrhal stage** (2 weeks): Nasal congestion, runny nose, low-grade fever, nonproductive cough. **Paroxysmal stage** (1–6 weeks): Severe "whooping" coughing spasms with thick sputum, especially at night. Infants may have apnea rather than whooping. **Convalescent stage** (up to 6 weeks): Gradual decrease in coughing. Treated with antibiotics. Use droplet precautions until 5 days after initiating antibiotics.
Influenza	Annual influenza	Abrupt fever, chills, aching, cough, runny nose, sore throat, and headache. Infants and young children: May have croup, conjunctivitis, nausea, vomiting, diarrhea, abdominal pain. Complications (most common in pediatric and geriatric patients): Otitis media, worsening of chronic lung conditions, pneumonia, myocarditis, encephalitis, Guillain-Barré syndrome, Reye's syndrome. Use droplet and contact precautions.
Mononucleosis	N/A	Fever (2–3 days), sore throat, swollen tonsils, lymphadenopathy, enlarged spleen and liver, fatigue, malaise. Infants and young children may be asymptomatic. Symptoms usually last 2–3 weeks, although weakness may persist for months. Complications (rare): Encephalitis, meningitis, Guillain-Barré syndrome, ruptured spleen, low platelet count. Use standard precautions.

Disease	Vaccine	Characteristics/Considerations
Herpes simplex 1	N/A	A blistering oral lesion or lesions on any other area of the skin. Cold sores typically occur at the border of the lip. Herpetic whitlow (infected finger) is from an infected child sucking a finger. Neonatal infection may be disseminated and may affect the liver, lungs, and brain. Herpetic gingivostomatitis syndrome includes fever, bilateral lymphadenopathy, and lesions in the mouth and tongue, progressing to open painful ulcers making swallowing difficult, so the patient drools. Symptoms usually last 1–2 weeks. Treatment is with acyclovir. Use standard precautions.
Hantavirus pulmonary syndrome	N/A	Hantavirus is transmitted through contact with the nesting material, feces, or urine of infected rodents or contaminated food. Initial symptoms are flu-like with fatigue, fever, and muscle aches. Half of those patients who are infected also experience headaches, chills, nausea and vomiting, diarrhea, and abdominal pain. Late symptoms occur within 4–10 days and include cough, shortness of breath, and a feeling of smothering progressing to pulmonary edema and respiratory failure. **Prehospital Interventions**: Use standard precautions, manage the airway/ventilation/intubation and supplemental oxygen as needed, provide an IV access line.
Rabies	Rabies vaccine (CDC recommends this vaccine only to those at high risk of exposure)	Viral disease with an incubation period of 30–90 days. It is transmitted through contact with the saliva of an infected animal (dog, cat, fox, skunk, raccoon, bat). The virus enters through open skin and travels along the nerves to the brain. Initial symptoms: Fever, chills, malaise, and pain at the bite site. Late: Anxiety, agitation, hallucinations, weakness, paralysis, hydrophobia, coma, respiratory failure, and death. **Prehospital Interventions**: Wash animal bites with soap and water and irrigate with povidone iodine. Notify the receiving facility of the possible need for rabies prophylaxis. Use standard and droplet precautions, provide supportive care, manage airway/ventilation/intubation/supplemental oxygen as needed, and provide an IV access line.

Endocrine Emergencies

ENDOCRINE SYSTEM ORGANS AND GLANDS

The endocrine system consists of the following organs and glands:

- **Hypothalamus**: Links the endocrine and nervous systems; produces hormones that are stored in the posterior lobe of the pituitary gland; stimulates the pituitary to release hormones
- **Pineal gland**: Secretes melatonin and dimethyltryptamine, which control sleep cycles and dreaming
- **Pituitary gland**: The posterior lobe secretes oxytocin (it stimulates uterine contractions/lactation) and vasopressin (aka antidiuretic hormone, which raises BP and promotes water reabsorption); the anterior lobe secretes hormones that control cell growth (somatotropin), body growth (growth hormone), release of hormones by the thyroid (thyrotropin), release of steroids from the adrenal glands (corticotropin), and reproductive functions (follicle-stimulating hormone and luteinizing hormone)
- **Thyroid gland**: Secretes hormones that control protein production, basal metabolic rate, and oxygen consumption (T3, T4, and calcitonin)
- **Parathyroid glands**: Secretes parathyroid hormone, which controls the use of calcium
- **Adrenal glands**: Produce cortisol (roles in metabolism), aldosterone (water and sodium levels), and androgens (male hormones)
- **Ovaries**: Secrete female hormones (estrogen and progesterone)
- **Testes**: Secrete androgens (testosterone)

> **Review Video: Endocrine System**
> Visit mometrix.com/academy and enter code: 678939

DIABETIC CONDITIONS

Diabetes mellitus is a group of metabolic disorders that involve hyperglycemia (increased blood glucose [sugar]) because of defective production and/or action of insulin. Insulin metabolizes glucose to produce energy as fuel for body cells.

- **Type 1**: Autoimmune destruction of beta cells in the pancreas results in no or deficient insulin production. Treatment is with insulin. Symptoms include rapid onset, increased thirst, frequent urination, increased hunger, delayed healing, weight loss, frequent infections, and blurred vision.
- **Type 2**: Insulin baseline may be normal or deficient, but there is no or an inadequate increase in response to a meal, so the glucose level rises but there is decreased uptake by the tissues. Insulin resistance occurs because there is decreased sensitivity to insulin by the tissues. Type 2 diabetes is often related to older age and obesity. Treatment is with oral diabetic agents. Symptoms include slow onset, increased thirst, increased urination, candidal (fungal) infections, delayed healing, and weight gain.
- **Gestational**: Beta cells in the pancreas are unable to produce adequate insulin during pregnancy, but normal production resumes after delivery. Treatment varies. Symptoms include increased thirst, urinary frequency, or sometimes no symptoms at all.

> **Review Video: Diabetes Mellitus**
> Visit mometrix.com/academy and enter code: 501396

HYPERGLYCEMIA AND DIABETIC KETOACIDOSIS

Hyperglycemia is high blood glucose (sugar) with a level >126 mg/dL after fasting for 8 hours or >180 mg/dL 2 hours after eating. Hyperglycemia may occur in undiagnosed diabetic patients, diabetic patients who have taken inadequate insulin, those who have eaten a diet too high in carbohydrates (sugars), or those who are ill, such as with an infection. It can also be induced by certain medications, such as steroids, statins, thiazide diuretics, and some antipsychotics. Initial signs include polyuria (increased urine), polyphagia (hunger), polydipsia (increased thirst), headaches, lethargy, fatigue, and blurred vision, but if the blood sugar is very high (>250 mg/dL), then patients may become increasingly somnolent, and he or she may develop **diabetic ketoacidosis** from the buildup of ketones as fat is broken down by the body for energy because sugar/glucose cannot be used. The patient may exhibit Kussmaul's breathing (fruity-smelling breath from ketones), lapse into a coma, and die if left untreated.

Prehospital Interventions: Question the patient about diabetes and the use of diabetes medications. Check the patient's blood sugar level, and monitor the vital signs and oxygen saturation. Manage the airway and assisted ventilation as needed, and provide an IV access line and crystalloid fluids and regular insulin if indicated. Rapid transport is required with altered levels of consciousness.

HYPERGLYCEMIC HYPEROSMOLAR NONKETOTIC SYNDROME (HHNS) OR COMA (HHNK)

Hyperglycemic hyperosmolar nonketotic syndrome (HHNS) or coma (HHNK) occurs in people without a history of diabetes or in people with mild type 2 diabetes but with insulin resistance resulting in persistent hyperglycemia, which causes osmotic diuresis. Fluid shifts from intracellular to extracellular spaces to maintain osmotic equilibrium, but the increased glycosuria and dehydration result in hypernatremia and increased osmolality (concentration). This condition is most common in persons 50–70 years old, and it often is precipitated by an acute illness such as a stroke, medications such as thiazides, or dialysis treatments. HHNS differs from ketoacidosis because although the insulin level is not adequate, it is high enough to prevent the breakdown of fat. Symptoms include polyuria, dehydration, hypotension, tachycardia, blood glucose >500 mg/dL, changes in mental status, hallucinations, seizures, and hemiparesis.

Prehospital Interventions: Question the patient about his or her history of diabetes and use of diabetes medications. Check the patient's blood sugar level, monitor the vital signs and oxygen saturation, and provide supportive care and an IV access line as needed. Rapid transport is needed for altered levels of consciousness.

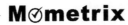

HYPOGLYCEMIA

Hypoglycemia (low blood sugar/glucose) is most often caused by an insulin reaction (too much insulin for the amount of glucose/sugar intake) or an overdose of oral diabetes medications, which stimulate the overproduction of insulin. Hypoglycemia may occur if patients took insulin but skipped a meal, vomited, or exercised too strenuously, depleting the body of sugar/glucose while insulin levels remain high. Increased insulin levels cause glucose levels to fall to ≤70 mg/dL, initially resulting in tremors, headache, blurred vision, dizziness, and pallor leading to confusion, bizarre behavior, lack of coordination, combative behavior, personality changes, tachycardia, and irregular heartbeat. Severe hypoglycemia may lead to seizures, coma, and death. Hypoglycemia is life threatening if untreated. Infants may have dehydration and seizures; geriatric patients may have dehydration and stroke.

Prehospital Interventions: Ask the patient about his or her diabetes status and use of diabetes medications. Check the patient's glucose level, and administer oral glucose tablets, one tablespoon of sugar, or a glass of orange juice if the patient is able to swallow. Provide rapid transport for altered levels of consciousness.

Psychiatric Conditions

BEHAVIORAL ALTERATIONS

Behavioral alterations may include agitation, anger, throwing temper tantrums (children), acting aggressively (adolescents/adult), exhibiting poor judgment, and acting inappropriately. **Behavioral alterations** may result from psychiatric disorders (e.g., depression, schizophrenia, bipolar disorder) and psychiatric medications as well as numerous other causes, including the following:

- Hypoglycemia/low blood sugar (insulin reaction)
- Lack of adequate oxygen interfering with brain function
- Shock (low BP; a rapid pulse results in inadequate blood supply to the brain)
- Mind-altering substances (cocaine, methamphetamine, LSD, Rohypnol [date-rape drug])
- Brain infection (meningitis, encephalitis, brain abscess)
- Seizure disorders (epilepsy, other causes of seizures)
- Poisoning/Overdose (lead poisoning, drug overdose)
- Malnutrition resulting in inadequate nourishment of brain tissue
- Substance abuse (drug or alcohol abuse/withdrawal)
- Heat extremes (hypothermia/hyperthermia)

Indications of being a danger to self or others include severe agitation, hallucinations, delusional thinking, paranoia, self-destructive behavior (e.g., cutting, drug/alcohol abuse, promiscuity, risk-taking activities), depression, and suicide attempts. A patient may pose a risk to others if he or she is behaving in a threatening or violent manner and has a weapon (e.g., gun, knife, baseball bat).

ASSESSMENT OF PSYCHIATRIC PATIENTS

Assessment of patients with psychological/psychiatric symptoms should begin with a history that includes the patient's age and cultural/spiritual background and whether the patient has experienced similar symptoms previously or has a history of a psychiatric disorder as well as any history of substance abuse. **Assessment** includes the following:

- **General appearance:** Note hygiene, grooming, appropriate dress, eye contact, unusual movements (twitching, posturing, repetitive movements), and the appearance and condition of the skin.
- **Speech**: Note speech cadence and abnormal word use, such as neologisms (invented words), clang associations (rhyming), word salad (string of random words), and associative looseness (ideas shifting from one to another).
- **Posture/Gait:** Note automatisms (purposeless behaviors, such as drumming fingers), slowed motions, waxy flexibility (maintaining an awkward position for extended periods of time), ability to walk, and abnormalities of gait.
- **Mental status**: Note the patient's state of being alert versus non-alert, responsive versus unresponsive, and coherent versus incoherent; clarity of ideas; suicidal ideation; and desire for self-harm.
- **Mood and affect**: Note facial expressions, expressed emotions, and affect (blunted, broad, flat, inappropriate, restricted).
- **Memory/Intellectual processes**: Note if memory and intellectual processes are intact or impaired. Is the patient disoriented and confused or alert and responsive?
- **Attention**: Note if the patient's attention is focused or unfocused.

ASSESSING FOR RISK OF SUICIDE

Suicidal ideation occurs frequently in those with mood disorders or depression (common in geriatric patients). Although females are more likely to attempt suicide, males actually successfully commit suicide three times more often, primarily because females tend to take overdoses from which they can be revived, whereas males choose more violent means (jumping from a high place, shooting, or hanging). This holds true for adolescents and adults. Risk factors include psychiatric disorders (schizophrenia, bipolar disorder, post-traumatic stress disorder [PTSD], and substance abuse), physical disorders (HIV/AIDS, diabetes, traumatic brain injury, spinal cord injury), and social problems (bullying). Passive suicidal ideation involves wishing to be dead or thinking about dying without making plans, whereas active suicidal ideation involves making plans. Patients at risk should be questioned about their feelings, problems, plans for suicide, and access to weapons. High-risk findings include the following:

- Violent suicide attempt (knives, gunshots) or access to a weapon
- History of a suicide attempt and a suicide attempt with a low chance of rescue
- Ongoing psychosis or disordered thinking
- Ongoing severe depression and feelings of helplessness
- Lack of a social support system

SCHIZOPHRENIA AND PSYCHOSIS

Schizophrenia, a thought disorder, causes psychotic episodes and distortion of reality and the inability to determine the line between fantasy and reality. The onset may be acute or more insidious. Symptoms are positive (delusions, hallucinations, disorganized or catatonic behavior, disorganized speech) or negative (flat affect/decreased emotional range, social isolation, poverty of speech, lack of interest and drive). Patients may have bizarre delusions (thought broadcasting) or hear voices (which they may try to drown out by turning the TV, radio, or music volume up loud). Patients may isolate themselves socially, exhibit poor hygiene, exhibit catatonia (a stiff, unmoving position), and have odd speech. Treatment is with typical and atypical antipsychotics and antidepressants (such as selective serotonin reuptake inhibitors [SSRIs]).

Psychosis is not a disease but a description of a condition and may apply to various diagnoses (such as schizophrenia and bipolar disease). Psychosis is characterized by marked derangement of the personality and a distorted view of reality. Patients may experience hallucinations (seeing/hearing something not present), delusions (false or distorted beliefs), and illusions (false impressions).

Prehospital Interventions: Provide supportive care.

DELIRIUM

Delirium is an acute sudden change in consciousness, characterized by reduced ability to focus or sustain attention, language and memory disturbance, disorientation, confusion, audiovisual hallucinations, sleep disturbance, and psychomotor activity disorder. **Delirium** differs from disorders with similar symptoms in that delirium is fluctuating. Delirium occurs in 10%–40% of hospitalized older adults and about 80% of patients who are terminally ill. Delirium may result from drugs such as anticholinergics and numerous conditions including infection, hypoxia, trauma, dementia, depression, vision and hearing loss, surgery, alcoholism, untreated pain, fluid/electrolyte imbalance, and malnutrition. Delirium increases the risks of morbidity and death, especially if untreated. Asking the patient to count backward from 20 to 1 and spell his or her first name backward can identify an attention deficit.

Prehospital Interventions: Ensure the patient's safety, manage the patient's airway, ventilation, and oxygen supplementation, and reorient the patient frequently.

AGITATED/EXCITED DELIRIUM

Patients with agitated/excited delirium are often very combative, aggressive, violent, and uncooperative, and they may exhibit shouting, threaten violence, and behave bizarrely. The patient may experience hallucinations, disorientation, paranoia, and panic. Patients may be exceptionally strong and seem insensitive to pain. They are often hyperthermic (high temperature). Agitated or excited delirium may be associated with hypoglycemia, brain damage, chemical imbalance, and substance abuse (methamphetamine, cocaine, phencyclidine [PCP, angel dust], and LSD). Patients often require restraints for their own or for others' safety, but they are at risk of death by asphyxiation or restraint (positional) because they fight desperately against the restraints.

Prehospital Interventions: The EMS provider should use active listening and try to establish rapport while assessing the patient's intellectual functioning, orientation, judgment and thought processes, language, mood, and appearance to determine if law enforcement or other assistance is needed. The patient may refuse care, but implied consent is legal for patients with abnormal behavior. The patient must be transported safely for treatment. The EMS provider should look for medications or drugs on site and take them to the receiving facility.

CALMING PATIENTS WITH BEHAVIORAL EMERGENCIES

Patients with **behavioral emergencies** are often agitated and may be confused, fearful, and/or aggressive, so the paramedic must remain calm and approach the patient slowly; remain at a safe distance; and avoid fast movements, threatening postures, or attempts at physical contact, acknowledging the patient's agitation and offering assistance ("I can see that you're upset, and I want to help") and maintaining eye contact (unless the person is violent and reacts aggressively). The EMT should encourage the patient to talk about what is causing the behavior and should answer questions honestly while avoiding threatening, arguing, or challenging the patient. If the patient is suffering hallucinations or delusional thinking, the EMT should avoid playing along ("I don't see what you do") but should also avoid contradicting the patient directly when responding. Family or friends may assist with intervention. The EMT should not leave the patient unattended and should try to lower distressing stimuli (such as lights and noise) and consider contacting law enforcement. Restraints should be avoided if possible.

RESTRAINTS

If a combative patient poses a risk to him- or herself or EMS personnel, **restraints** may be necessary to safely assess, treat, and transport the patient, keeping in mind that the altered state of consciousness may result from drug or alcohol use; traumatic injury; or from a mental or physical disorder, such as schizophrenia, dementia, or hypoglycemia (insulin reaction). Protocols for use of restraints must be followed, and restraints should be applied under medical direction. If possible, the police should be present and there should be one EMS personnel for each limb, staying beyond the limb's range of motion until ready to secure the limb, with one EMT talking to the patient and explaining the procedure. The EMT should avoid unnecessary force, which may result in increased combativeness and injury to the patient or others. Patients should not be restrained in the prone (face-down) position. Documentation must include the reason for restraining the patient, the time, and the method of restraint.

TYPES OF RESTRAINTS

Patients needing restraints are often agitated, confused, and refuse care, but implied consent is legal for patients with abnormal behavior. **Types of restraints** include the following:

- **Verbal:** Try to calm the patient while being firm.
- **Nonverbal:** Use body language and a show of force (with a number of EMS personnel being present) to convince the patient.
- **Physical:** Use standard precautions; one person is assigned to each limb, while a fifth person reassures and tries to calm the patient. Apply multiple restraints as necessary, including across the trunk, being careful not to restrict the patient's breathing.
- **Chemical:** Use as a last resort (usually after physical restraints). Includes benzodiazepines (lorazepam) and neuroleptics (haloperidol).
- **Tasers/electrical stun guns:** These may be used by law enforcement to subdue a severely agitated patient. They may cause burns, dart injuries, fall injuries, or cardiac arrest. Stun guns require direct contact, but Tasers may be shot from 20 feet away.

Document the reason for restraint, the types of restraints, the restraint technique, and the time the patient is restrained. Monitor the patient's condition continuously, including the heart rate, airway, ventilation, oxygen supplementation, and circulation.

TYPES OF PHYSICAL RESTRAINTS

Common types of physical restraints include the following:

- **Soft:** Padded cuffs (often leather) that fasten about the wrists and ankles and are attached to a long board. These are the most commonly used restraints.
- **Stretcher/Spinal board straps:** These may be strapped across the chest (not too tight), abdomen, or legs to help restrict movement.
- **Long board/Spinal board:** Patient should be restrained to the long board and then placed on a wheeled stretcher and never tied to or fastened to the stretcher.
- **Spit sock:** This is a hood that fits over the patient's head to prevent him or her from biting or spitting.
- **Cervical collar:** This is used to protect the patient's cervical spine and to prevent him or her from biting.

The EMT should not place the patient in handcuffs or hard plastic ties. If these were placed on a patient by a law enforcement officer and must stay in place, such as with a criminal suspect or an extremely violent patient, then a law enforcement officer must stay with the patient at all times.

Toxicology

ROUTES OF POISONING

Routes of poisoning include:

- **Ingestion**: Drugs, overdose, toxic/caustic liquids (bleach, cleaning solution, antifreeze, gasoline), mouse/rat poison, pesticides, some plants, and alcohol. There is a wide range of symptoms, depending on the substance: anaphylaxis, lethargy, constricted pupils, mouth burns, nausea and vomiting, pain, diarrhea, difficulty breathing, confusion, seizures, and coma. (Toddlers are particularly at risk.)
- **Inhalation**: Toxic gases, smoke, hair spray, carbon monoxide, chlorine, halogens. Symptoms include difficulty breathing, lethargy, confusion, nausea, vomiting, headache, cyanosis, seizures, slurred speech, and coma.
- **Injection**: Heroin, morphine, drug overdose. Symptoms include local irritation, lethargy, confusion, slurred speech, nausea, vomiting, difficulty breathing, seizures, and coma. (Adolescents are prone to experimentation with drugs.)
- **Absorption**: Cleaning products, various chemicals. Symptoms include local irritation, anaphylaxis, burns, tissue damage, rash, nausea, vomiting, shortness of breath, and confusion.

Prehospital Interventions: Treatment varies according to the severity. Contact a poison control center if necessary, provide supportive care, remove the substance residue from the patient's mouth, place the patient in the recovery position, manage the patient's airway/ventilation/oxygen supplementation, provide CPR as necessary, induce vomiting or administer activated charcoal only if advised by the poison control center or another expert, and provide rapid transport. If the contamination is by inhalation, remove the patient from the source as soon as possible. If the contamination is by absorption, remove the contaminated clothes, wash the patient's skin with large amounts of soap and water, and flush the affected eyes with water or NS.

NERVE AGENTS/CHOLINERGICS

Nerve agents/cholinergics are toxic chemicals (organophosphates) that damage the nervous system and bodily functions, leading to death in a short time. Nerve agents include tabun (GA), sarin (GB), soman (GD), and VX, and they are used in terrorist attacks. GA, BG, and GD persist in the environment for 10 minutes to 24 hours during the summer and 2 hours to 3 days during the winter (cold weather), and they have very fast action. VX persists longer in the environment and is more lethal. Symptoms of exposure (gas/aerosol) include salivation, lacrimation, urination, defecation, GI upset, and emesis; runny nose; pupil contraction; vision impairment; slurred speech; chest pain; hallucinations; respiratory distress; and coma. High doses may cause immediate seizures and death.

Prehospital Interventions: Move away from the area quickly or shelter in place, remove the patient's clothing, and wash the patient's body with large amounts of soap and water. Use an autoinjector for atropine and pralidoxime (separate injections [Mark I] or combined dose [DuoDote]), unless there is only mild tearing or a runny nose, and use diazepam for seizures. Provide airway/ventilation/oxygen supplementation and circulation support.

CARBON MONOXIDE POISONING

Carbon monoxide poisoning occurs when people breathe in carbon monoxide, usually related to industrial or household accidents or suicide attempts. Carbon monoxide binds to hemoglobin 200 times more readily than oxygen, and once the carbon monoxide binds to hemoglobin (creating carboxyhemoglobin), the hemoglobin can no longer bind to or transport oxygen, resulting in hypoxemia. Symptoms vary depending on the percentage of saturation with carbon monoxide. At 10%, patients may complain of headache and nausea. At >20%, a patient becomes increasingly weak and confused with alterations in mental status. At >30%, a patient may have dyspnea, chest pain, and increased confusion. When the level continues to increase, a patient may experience seizures, coma, and death. The patient's skin color may be cyanotic, pink, or bright cherry red (but this is not a reliable sign).

It is critical to note that pulse oximetry is not an accurate measure of oxygen saturation in patients with carbon monoxide poisoning because the technology cannot differentiate between oxygen and carbon monoxide binding to the blood.

Prehospital Interventions: Administer 100% oxygen with a nonrebreather mask and transport.

POISON CONTROL RESOURCES

The **National Capital Poison Center** provides a website with an online tool (called webPOISONCONTROL) and a telephone number (800-222-1222) for people who swallow or come into contact (absorbed, inhaled, or injected) with toxic substances.

- **webPOISONCONTROL** can be used for patients (ages 6 months to 79 years and nonpregnant women) who are asymptomatic and unintentionally came into contact with a single drug or medication, household product, or berries over a short period of time (minutes to a few hours) but are otherwise healthy.
- **Telephone contact** is used for all other situations, including a patient with symptoms, pregnant women, non-swallowing contact, those aged <6 months or >79, or those who swallowed materials or substances other than those listed for online assistance. Telephone contact can be made for any poisoning if it is preferred to online assistance.

This service is free and usually requires about 3 minutes for a response. When calling, be prepared to describe the substance (include the product name and dosage for medications), amount swallowed, age of patient, weight of patient, time since exposure, and the patient's ZIP Code and email address. If unsure of the amount of poison or the weight of the victim, estimates are acceptable.

AGE-RELATED CONCERNS RELATED TO TOXICOLOGY

Age-related concerns related to toxicology include the following:

- **Toddlers** are at risk of ingestion of toxic substances because their taste buds are not yet fully developed and this allows them to drink foul-tasting substances, such as cleaning supplies, which may be kept under a sink where a child has easy access if the cabinet is not secured. Household substances that pose a substantial risk include perfumes, cosmetics, and alcohol. Toddlers may also ingest unsecured medications.
- **Adolescents**, who often experiment with drugs and alcohol, are at risk from alcohol poisoning and overdose or severe reaction to illicit drugs. Additionally, adolescents often attempt suicide with acetaminophen (Tylenol), sometimes to gain attention, without realizing that it can cause liver failure and death even after resuscitation.
- **Geriatric patients** are most at risk from medication errors, such as taking the wrong medication, taking medications belonging to friends or family, or taking the wrong dose of a medication.

SUBSTANCE ABUSE

Many people with substance abuse (alcohol or drugs) are reluctant to disclose this information. Common agents include:

- Cannabis (marijuana)
- Hallucinogens (LSD)
- Stimulants (cocaine, methamphetamine)
- Barbiturates (secobarbital [Seconal] amobarbital [Amytal])
- Sedatives (zolpidem [Ambien], eszopiclone [Lunesta])
- Hypnotics/benzodiazepines (alprazolam [Xanax], diazepam [Valium]
- Lorazepam [Ativan])
- Opiates (heroin, morphine, fentanyl, oxycodone, hydrocodone)

A number of indicators are suggestive of **substance abuse**.

Physical Signs

- Needle tracks on arms or legs
- Burns on fingers or lips
- Pupils abnormally dilated or constricted, eyes watery
- Slurring of speech, slow speech
- Lack of coordination, instability of gait
- Tremors
- Sniffing repeatedly, nasal irritation
- Persistent cough
- Weight loss
- Dysrhythmias (abnormal pulse)
- Pallor, puffiness of face

Other Signs

- Odor of alcohol/marijuana on clothing or breath
- Labile emotions, including mood swings, agitation, and anger
- Inappropriate, impulsive, and/or risky behavior
- Lying
- Missing appointments
- Difficulty concentrating/short-term memory loss, disoriented/confused
- Blackouts
- Insomnia or excessive sleeping
- Lack of personal hygiene

Ethanol (Alcohol) Abuse and Withdrawal

Ethanol (the alcohol that is found in alcoholic beverages, flavorings, and some medications) is a multisystem toxin and CNS depressant. It is often the drug of choice of teenagers, young adults, and those >60 years old. **Ethanol overdose** affects the CNS and other organs. If patients are easily aroused, they can usually safely sleep off the effects, but if a patient is semiconscious or unconscious, emergency medical treatment is needed. Young children frequently ingest alcohol in products such as perfumes and cleaning solutions, which are often more toxic than alcoholic beverages.

Infants/Young Children

- Seizures, coma, death
- Respiratory depression and hypoxia
- Hypoglycemia (especially infants and toddlers)
- Hypothermia

Teenagers/Adults

- Altered mental status, coma, circulatory collapse, death
- Hypotension, bradycardia with arrhythmias
- Respiratory depression and hypoxia
- Cold, clammy skin or flushed skin
- Acute pancreatitis/abdominal pain

Chronic abuse of ethanol (alcoholism) is associated with **alcohol withdrawal syndrome** (delirium tremens) with abrupt cessation of alcohol intake, resulting in hallucinations, tachycardia, diaphoresis, sometimes psychotic behavior, and a high mortality rate.

Prehospital Interventions: Manage the patient's airway, ventilation, and oxygen supplementation and provide CPR if necessary, maintain body temperature, and reduce noise/light.

Hematologic Emergencies

COMPONENTS OF THE BLOOD

Blood cells are produced in the bone marrow. Blood is a viscous, dark-red fluid comprised of cells, gases, and plasma. Blood components include the following:

- **Erythrocytes** (red blood cells [RBCs]): RBCs carry hemoglobin, which transports oxygen. If the RBC count is low (such as from blood loss) or the oxygen-carrying capacity is impaired (such as with anemia), the patient may experience hypoxemia (low oxygen). The life cycle of RBCs is normally 120 days.
- **Leukocytes** (white blood cells [WBCs]): WBCs defend the body against invading organisms (viruses, bacteria, fungi, and parasites), and in the bloodstream and tissues they respond to allergies. WBCs include lymphocytes (B, T, natural killer, and null cells), monocytes, eosinophils, basophils, and neutrophils.
- **Thrombocytes** (platelets): Platelets release clotting factors and have an active role in forming blood clots.
- **Plasma** (55% of blood): Plasma carries water, proteins, electrolytes, lipids (fats), blood cells, and glucose as well as clotting factors.

The primary blood types are A, B, AB, and O. Blood is either Rh– or RH+, and patients must receive transfusions of blood that are type and Rh compatible.

HEMATOLOGICAL CONDITIONS

Hematological conditions include:

- **Anemia**: Anemia occurs when there are deficient numbers of RBCs or the hemoglobin doesn't bind to sufficient oxygen to meet body demands. Anemia results in a decrease in oxygen transportation and decreased perfusion throughout the body, causing the heart to compensate by increasing cardiac output. The types include iron-deficiency (inadequate iron), blood-loss, hemolytic (red cells destroyed), aplastic (bone marrow damaged), and pernicious (vitamin B_{12} deficiency) anemia.
- **Leukopenia**: A low WBC count (<4000) makes the patient vulnerable to infection. Causes include chemotherapy, autoimmune disorders, cancer, viral infections, medications (such as antibiotics), radiation, HIV/AIDS, and TB.
- **Lymphomas**: Cancer of the lymphocytes (the WBCs involved in the immune response). Two main types are Hodgkin's and non-Hodgkin's lymphoma.
- **Polycythemia**: Excessive RBC count, resulting in viscous (thick) blood and an increased risk of clots.
- **Multiple myeloma**: Cancer of the plasma cells, resulting in tumor in the bone marrow, bone pain, anemia, kidney failure, and infection.
- **Thrombocytopenia**: Low platelet count, increasing the risk of bruising and bleeding.

SICKLE CELL DISEASE

Sickle cell disease is a recessive genetic disorder of chromosome 11, causing hemoglobin to be defective so that the red blood cells (RBCs) are sickle-shaped and inflexible, resulting in their accumulating in small vessels and causing painful blockages. Although normal RBCs survive for 120 days, sickled blood cells may survive only 10–20 days, stressing the bone marrow that can't produce RBCs fast enough and resulting in anemia. Different types of **crises** occur (aplastic, hemolytic, vaso-occlusive, and sequestering), which can cause infarctions in organs, severe pain, damage to organs, and rapid enlargement of the liver and spleen. Vaso-occlusive crisis is common in adolescents and adults, and it can be triggered by sickness, stress, dehydration, temperature changes, and high altitude. Young children are prone to splenic sequestration (RBCs trapped in the spleen, causing it to enlarge and sometimes rupture), which is characterized by pain in the left abdomen.

Prehospital Interventions: Manage the patient's airway, ventilation, and oxygen supplementation and circulation, provide emotional support, and provide rapid transport for severe symptoms.

CLOTTING DISORDERS

Clotting disorders include the following:

- **Hemophilia** is an inherited disorder in which the person lacks adequate clotting factors, which results in bleeding with trauma, bruising, spontaneous hemorrhage (often in the joints), and epistaxis. There are three primary types: A (80–90%), B, and C.
- **Disseminated intravascular coagulation (DIC)** (consumption coagulopathy) is a secondary disorder that is triggered by another event, such as trauma, congenital heart disease, necrotizing enterocolitis, sepsis, and severe viral infections. DIC triggers coagulation (clotting) and hemorrhage through a complex series of events, with clotting and hemorrhage occurring simultaneously, putting the patient at risk of death.
- **Von Willebrand's disease** is a group of congenital bleeding disorders (inherited from either parent) affecting 1-2% of the population, associated with deficiency or lack of von Willebrand factor (vWF), a glycoprotein.

Prehospital Interventions: Monitor for signs of bleeding, and manage the patient's airway/ventilation/oxygen supplementation. Provide rapid transport for hemorrhage or acute blood loss resulting in hypotension.

Genitourinary Emergencies

COMPONENTS OF THE GENITOURINARY SYSTEM

The **genitourinary system** encompasses the organs of the urinary system and the organs of the reproductive system. The **urinary system** is comprised of two kidneys (which are located in the right and left flank areas) that filter the blood of toxins and excess fluid, creating urine. The ureters carry the urine to the bladder where urine is stored, and the urethra carries the urine from the bladder to the external meatus (opening) during urination. The male urethra is about 18-20 cm long, while the female urethra is only 3-4 cm long, placing females at more at risk for ascending infections.

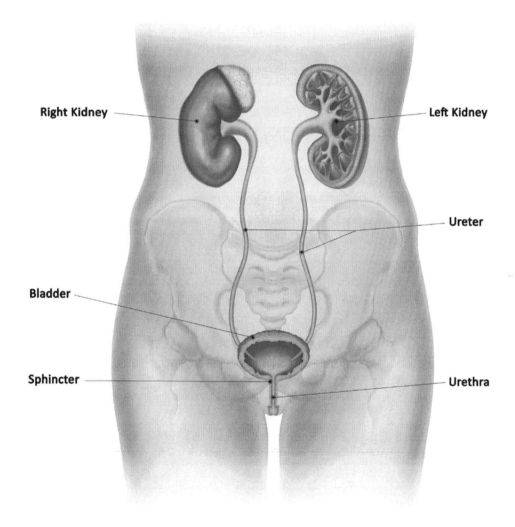

> **Review Video: Urinary System**
> Visit mometrix.com/academy and enter code: 601053

The **male reproductive system** includes the scrotum, two testes, the epididymis, spermatic cords and vas deferens, seminal vesicles, ejaculatory duct, prostate, urethra, Cowper's glands, and penis. The **female reproductive system** includes the ovaries, fallopian tubes, uterus, and vagina as well as the breasts.

> **Review Video: Reproductive Systems**
> Visit mometrix.com/academy and enter code: 505450

RENAL AND URINARY CALCULI

Renal (kidney) and urinary calculi (stones) occur frequently, more commonly in males, and they can be related to diseases (hyperparathyroidism, renal tubular acidosis, and gout) and lifestyle factors, such as sedentary work. Their incidence is highest between ages 35 and 45. Additionally, some medications can precipitate calculi. Calculi can form at any age, most are composed of calcium, and can range in size from very tiny to >6 mm. Stones of <4 mm can usually pass in the urine easily.

Symptoms occur with obstruction and are usually of sudden onset and acute.

- Severe flank pain radiating to the abdomen and labia or testicle on the same side as the stone (adolescents and adults), abdominal or pelvic pain (young children)
- Nausea and vomiting
- Diaphoresis
- Hematuria (blood in urine)

Prehospital Interventions:

- Analgesia: Opiates and NSAIDs as needed (per protocol)
- Provide supplemental oxygen if needed
- Start an IV access line and give fluids if indicated
- Transport

RENAL FAILURE

Acute renal failure is an abrupt and almost complete failure of kidney function, occurring over a period of hours or days. It most commonly occurs in hospitalized patients, but it may occur in others as well. Causes include MI, heart failure, sepsis, anaphylaxis, burns, trauma, infections, transfusion reactions, medications (NSAIDs and ACE inhibitors), and obstruction. Symptoms include reduced or absent urinary output, increased nocturia (nighttime urination), altered mental status, tinnitus, a metallic taste in the mouth, tremors, seizures, flank pain, abdominal pain, hypertension, increased bruising.

Chronic renal failure occurs after years of disease that damages the kidneys, often being essentially asymptomatic until the damage is severe. Early symptoms may include anorexia, general malaise, headaches, itching, and weight loss. Later symptoms include fluid retention (pulmonary edema, peripheral edema, ascites), headache, bruising, dry skin, muscle cramping, bone pain, weakness, breath odor, excessive thirst, frequent hiccups, dyspnea, vomiting (especially in the morning), and hypertension.

Prehospital Interventions: Manage the patient's airway/ventilation/oxygen, provide an IV access line (if the patient is hypotensive or if there is evidence of pulmonary edema), and transport.

END-STAGE RENAL DISEASE (ESRD)

Acute and chronic renal failure may progress to **end-stage renal disease (ESRD)** when the kidneys are no longer able to function and the patient needs dialysis or a kidney transplant. The patient may develop uremic syndrome, which results in decreased production of red blood cells and platelets, electrolyte imbalances, bone disease, multiple endocrine disorders, cardiac problems (especially congestive heart failure), anorexia, and malnutrition. Symptoms include altered mental status, hallucinations, and confusion from the accumulation of waste products in the blood; increasing edema and shortness of breath from accumulated fluids; chest and bone pain; severe pruritus; nausea, vomiting, and diarrhea; tremors, muscle twitching, and seizures; and increased bruising and discoloration of the skin.

> **Review Video: End Stage Renal Disease**
> Visit mometrix.com/academy and enter code: 869617

Prehospital Interventions: Manage the patient's airway/ventilation/oxygen, start an IV access line (if the patient is hypotensive or if there is evidence of pulmonary edema), and transport.

MANAGEMENT

HEMODIALYSIS

Hemodialysis is used primarily for those who have progressed from renal insufficiency to uremia with end-stage renal (kidney) disease (ESRD). With hemodialysis, blood is circulated outside of the body through a dialyzer (a synthetic semipermeable membrane), which filters the blood and removes waste products and excess fluids. A vascular access device, such as a catheter, fistula, or graft, must be established for hemodialysis, with fistulas and grafts usually placed in an arm and a catheter placed in the upper chest (into the superior vena cava). Tubing from the dialysis machine attaches to the access device for treatments, which are usually done for 4 hours three times weekly. Emergent conditions include low BP, nausea/vomiting, irregular pulse, cardiac arrest, bleeding from the access site, and difficulty breathing. Missed treatments may result in electrolyte excess, weakness, and pulmonary edema.

Prehospital Interventions: Manage the patient's airway/ventilation/oxygen supplementation, apply pressure to stop any bleeding, position the patient flat if he or she is in shock, and position upright if there is difficulty breathing. Provide an IV access, but avoid placing the IV and measuring the BP on the arm with the access site.

PERITONEAL DIALYSIS

Peritoneal dialysis is used to remove waste products and excess fluids from those with ESRD. A catheter is placed into the peritoneal cavity of the abdomen. The peritoneum comprises the visceral peritoneum (the lining of the gut and other viscera), which makes up about 80% of the total peritoneal surface area, and the parietal perineum (lining the abdominal cavity), which is the most important for peritoneal dialysis. A dialysate solution is instilled (usually about 2 L for adults but less for children, taking about 10 minutes) through the catheter, the catheter is clamped, and the solution is left in place for 3–6 hours (dwell time). The solution is then drained (usually for about 20 minutes), and the process is repeated with new dialysate. Peritoneal dialysis increases the risk of obesity, peritonitis, hernia, malnutrition, hypertriglyceridemia, and back pain. Obesity, older adulthood, and lack of social support are contraindications for peritoneal dialysis.

Prehospital Interventions: Manage the patient's airway/ventilation/oxygen supplementation, use contact precautions if there is purulent drainage from the catheter site, and position the patient for comfort.

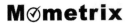

URINARY CATHETER MANAGEMENT

A **urinary catheter** is inserted through the urethra and into the bladder to drain urine. Straight catheterizations are done with sterile catheters periodically to empty the bladder or to relieve urinary retention, whereas retention catheters (Foley) have a balloon that inflates to keep the catheter in place for continuous drainage. Foley catheters may be indicated for patients with neuromuscular disorders, incontinence, urinary retention, dementia, or urinary disorders. Catheters may also be inserted suprapubically (above the pubis bone) directly into the bladder, especially for males with long-term catheterization. Urinary collection bags should be kept below the level of the bladder, and the tubing is secured so that the catheter is not inadvertently pulled out, causing trauma to the urethra, especially in males. Thick, cloudy urine may indicate infection. Scant urine and lower abdominal pain/distension may indicate blockage of the catheter. Milking the catheter may help relieve a blockage. When removing a Foley catheter, the balloon must first be deflated.

Prehospital Interventions: Provide supportive care, start an IV access line, and give fluids to keep the vein open if there is severe abdominal pain.

Eyes

MANUAL EYE IRRIGATION

Manual eye irrigation is indicated to remove foreign bodies, exudate, and chemicals from the eye. With chemicals, continuous irrigation with copious amounts of fluids (NS or lactated ringers ideally, though tap water may be used in emergent situations) should be carried out for at least 15 minutes. Procedure:

1. If possible, remove contact lenses, but with chemical burns, leave lenses in place to avoid delay unless the eye is swelling rapidly. Change gloves after removing contact lenses.
2. Place absorbent pads under the face and place a curved kidney-shaped basin below cheek on affected side.
3. Wipe secretions or visible reside (inner canthus to outer) from eyelids with gauze moistened with NS.
4. Retract upper and lower eyelids to expose conjunctival sacs.
5. Irrigate from inner canthus (using a dropper, IV tubing, or irrigation syringe), toward the outer canthus, ensuring that the tip remains 1 inch from inner canthus.
6. Ask the patient to look upward and continue irrigation.
7. Allow the patient to periodically blink.
8. When completed, blot moisture and assess eye for reactivity, visual acuity, and comfort.

Nose

NOSEBLEED (EPISTAXIS)

Recurrent nosebleed (epistaxis) is common in young children (ages 2–10), especially boys, and it is often related to nose picking, dry climate, trauma, or central heating. Its incidence also increases between 50 and 80 years of age and may be associated with NSAIDs, hypertension, and anticoagulants. Patients abusing cocaine may suffer nosebleeds because of damage to the mucosa. The anterior nares have plentiful blood vessels and may bleed easily, usually from one nostril. Bleeding in the posterior nares is more dangerous and can result in considerable blood loss. Blood may flow through both nostrils or backward into the throat, and the person may swallow and vomit blood. The blood may block the airway in unconscious patients

Prehospital Interventions: Have the patient sit in an upright position, leaning forward so blood doesn't flow down the throat. Have the patient pinch the nostrils together firmly for at least 10 minutes. Advise the patient to avoid sniffing or blowing the nose.

Obstetric Emergencies

PREMONITORY SIGNS OF LABOR

Premonitory signs of labor include:

- **Lightening**: As the fetal head engages and moves toward the birth canal, the fundal pressure on the diaphragm lessens, so the mother can breathe more easily, but pressure in the pelvic area increases, causing urinary frequency. The lower abdomen may protrude more than previously. Increased circulatory impairment may cause venous stasis and ankle edema as well as increased vaginal secretions as the vaginal mucous membranes become congested. Pressure on the nerves may result in leg cramps or increased pelvic, back and leg pain.
- **Braxton Hicks (BH)**: BH contractions are short in duration, occur at irregular intervals in the lower abdomen, and do not change the cervix. They are often relieved by activity or mild analgesia. The intensity and frequency of BH contractions often increase immediately prior to the onset of true labor.
- **Cervical changes**: The cervix ripens (softens) to allow for effacement (thinning) and dilation.
- **Bloody show**: A mucous plug from pooled secretions forms at the opening of the cervical canal during pregnancy; when the cervix begins to efface, this mucous plug is expelled, exposing capillary vessels that bleed. Bloody show typically appears as pink mucus and usually occurs within 24 to 48 hours of the onset of labor.
- **Ruptured membranes**: Rupture of the membranes occurs in about 12% of women prior to the onset of labor, which usually then occurs within 24 hours. Before rupture, the membranes typically bulge through the dilating cervix; fluid comes in a gush, although it may come in smaller spurts in some cases. If the membranes rupture before engagement of the fetal head, the umbilical cord may prolapse with the fluid, increasing the risk to the fetus, so mothers should always seek medical attention after rupture. If the mother is at term and labor does not start within 24 hours of rupture, labor may be induced.

STAGES OF LABOR

The stages of labor proceed as follows:

- **First stage (dilation stage)**: Consists of three phases
  - **Latent phase**: The cervix begins to dilate from 0-3 cm; contractions are mild to moderate and occur every 3-30 minutes and are of short duration.
  - **Active phase**: The cervix dilates from 4-7 cm; contractions are every 1-5 minutes, lasting 20-40 seconds. Pain is increased.
  - **Transitional phase**: The cervix dilates from 8-10 cm; contractions come every 1.5-2.0 minutes, lasting 60-90 seconds. There is increased pain, hyperventilation, crying, moaning, vomiting, and rectal pressure.
- **Second stage (expulsion stage)**: Starts when the cervix is fully dilated and ends with delivery of the baby. The patient feels an uncontrollable urge to push, the perineum begins to bulge, and the fetal head crowns as the mother begins to bear down and birth is imminent. Pressure on the rectum and anus may cause stool to be expelled. Birth occurs head first if it is a normal delivery, feet first if it is a breech delivery.
- **Third stage (placental stage)**: Delivery of the placenta should occur 5-30 minutes after birth. There are two phases: placental separation and placental expulsion. Normal blood loss as a result of placental separation is 300-500 mL. Retained placenta may occur if more than 30 minutes elapse.
- **Fourth stage**: The period of 1-4 hours after birth, which involves 250-400 mL blood loss, moderate hypotension (low BP), and tachycardia (rapid pulse).

ANATOMICAL STRUCTURES OF PREGNANCY

The anatomical structures involved with pregnancy and fetal development are contained within the female **uterus** (womb). The **placenta** is attached to the walls of the uterus; it includes the **umbilical cord**, which provides blood, nutrients, and oxygen to the fetus. The fetus is inside an **amniotic sac**, which contains amniotic fluid that cushions the fetus. The opening to the uterus is the **cervix**, which thins and dilates for delivery. The cervix opens into the **vagina**, which acts as the birth canal.

VAGINAL BLEEDING DURING PREGNANCY

Vaginal bleeding may occur during any part of a pregnancy and may be related to any of the structures within the uterus. Vaginal bleeding during the **first trimester** of pregnancy may indicate spontaneous abortion, ectopic pregnancy, or infection, although light occasional spotting may be normal. All vaginal bleeding during pregnancy should be assessed by a physician, and a large amount of bleeding may indicate a medical emergency. Bloody show near term may indicate that delivery is near.

Prehospital Interventions: Use standard precautions and position the patient on her left side. Place a sanitary pad over the vaginal opening and save any soaked pads in a plastic bag so the physician can estimate the amount of blood loss. Manage the patient's airway, ventilation, and oxygen supplementation and provide emotional support. Provide an IV access line and fluids if indicated.

DELIVERY OF A NEWBORN

If the fetal head is obvious at the vaginal opening (crowning), delivery is imminent. Steps to delivery include the following:

1. Wash hands and don PPE for standard precautions and obtain an OB kit and supplies.
2. Position the patient on her back with hips and knees flexed, feet flat on the stretcher, and legs apart.
3. Position one person at the mother's head to support and care for the mother, while the other person delivers the baby.
4. Provide oxygen to the mother, and if time allows, provide an IV access line and NS, cardiac monitoring, and analgesia as needed.
5. As the infant's head is crowning, support the perineum with the palm of your hand, also supporting the baby's head as it delivers.
6. Palpate the neck to determine if the umbilical cord has wrapped around the neck. If there is a nuchal cord, carefully attempt to slip it over the infant's head.
7. Once the body delivers, make note of the time of birth.
8. If the infant is not vigorous, stimulate by drying with a towel, and possibly suctioning the mouth and nose with a bulb syringe. Blow-by oxygen or bag-mask ventilation is utilized if the infant is not breathing.
9. If the infant is stable, place the baby skin to skin on mom's chest.
10. After about 2 minutes, place a cord clamp about 4 cm from the neonate's abdomen, and another cord clamp or hemostat a few centimeters down, then cut the cord in between the clamps.
11. Monitor the baby and assign an Apgar score at one and five minutes after birth.
12. Placental separation and delivery usually occur within 10-20 minutes after birth. Never pull on the umbilical cord as it may cause uterine inversion or placental tearing.
13. Place a sanitary pad over the vaginal opening to contain any bleeding. Observe for hemorrhage.
14. The uterus should be massaged to promote contractions and control excessive bleeding.

INITIAL ASSESSMENT OF THE PREGNANT PATIENT

Initial assessment of a pregnant patient should determine if the patient's emergency is related to the pregnancy (bleeding, cramping, pain, contractions), to an accident (fall or other injury), or to an unrelated illness:

- Assess patient's vital signs, including oxygen saturation. Monitor ECG.
- Assess pain using the 1-10 numeric scale.
- Determine the patient's week of gestation, singleton vs multiples, gravida, and parity.
- Determine if the patient has had prenatal care.
- If the patient is having contractions, determine the onset, frequency, and duration.
- If the patient is bleeding, determine if it is associated with trauma and estimate the amount, observe the character (dark, bright, scant, flowing, massive), and ask patient about onset and number of pads used in an hour.
- If BP is elevated, ask the patient about headaches, weight gain, seizures, and visual disturbances as these may indicate preeclampsia.
- If patient has supine hypotension, position patient on the left side with a blanket or roll under the left hip.
- Ask about medications including illegal drugs and history of substance abuse.

SPONTANEOUS AND ELECTIVE ABORTION

Spontaneous abortion: The unplanned loss of pregnancy at or before 20 weeks may result from trauma, fetal abnormality, or another cause. Indications include vaginal bleeding (mild to severe) and contractions. The patient may be very emotionally upset.

Prehospital Interventions: Use the term *miscarriage* rather than *abortion*, which has negative connotations for many. Gather any products of conception in a plastic bag to take to the hospital. Provide supportive care. Place a sanitary pad over the vagina. Provide reassurance and emotional support.

Elective abortion: Planned loss of pregnancy at or before 20 weeks per surgical procedure or abortion pills (during the first 10 weeks). Patients may develop bleeding after surgery or as the fetus is expelled.

Prehospital Interventions: Gather any products of conception in a plastic bag to take to the hospital, provide supportive care, place a sanitary pad over the vagina, and provide reassurance and emotional support.

ECTOPIC PREGNANCY

Ectopic pregnancy: Pregnancy in which the egg fertilizes and attaches outside of the uterus (usually in the fallopian tubes), resulting in abdominal pain, absent menstrual periods, and vaginal bleeding. There is a risk of the fallopian tube rupturing, resulting in internal hemorrhage, which is a life-threatening emergency.

Prehospital Interventions: As above. In the case of a rupture, start an IV and provide fluids. Monitor vital signs and level of consciousness. This patient will be rushed in for immediate surgery.

DELIVERY OF THE PRETERM INFANT

A **preterm** infant is one born prior to 37 weeks gestational age. In the United States, preterm birth is the most important factor influencing infant mortality, accounting for 75-80% of all neonatal morbidity and mortality. Preterm birth is often associated with comorbidities. The original cause of the preterm birth (such as maternal infection) may also play an integral role in the likely health problems associated with the infant's prematurity. Findings may include the following:

- Respiratory distress syndrome because of inadequate surfactant production (hyaline membrane disease)
- Hypothermia because of inadequate subcutaneous fat, small amounts of brown fat, and large skin surface area to mass ratio
- Hypoglycemia secondary to poor nutritional intake, poor nutritional stores, and increased glucose consumption associated with sepsis
- Skin trauma or infection secondary to fragile, transparent, immature skin with less subcutaneous fat
- Periods of apnea because of an immature respiratory center in the brain
- Intraventricular hemorrhage
- Large trunk and short extremities

Prehospital Interventions: Attempt resuscitation with signs of life, suction, ventilate/oxygenate, give compressions if indicated, administer epinephrine for bradycardia, and maintain body temperature.

COMPLICATIONS OF PREGNANCY AND LABOR

Complication	Characteristic	Prehospital Interventions
Preterm labor	Labor between weeks 20 and 37 weeks; presents a risk to the fetus.	Provide supportive care in the left lateral position. Manage the patient's airway, ventilation, and oxygen supplementation (100%). Transport rapidly if there is severe bleeding or a risk of imminent preterm delivery. Start an IV access line and give NS for placental abruption.
Premature rupture of membranes	Membranes rupture before the onset of labor; this may lead to preterm labor and risk to the fetus.	
Substance abuse	May result in damage to the fetus and preterm labor. Many drugs restrict blood flow to the fetus, resulting in growth restriction and low oxygen. Some drugs, such as cocaine, affect the fetal nervous system. Sudden withdrawal of opiates may trigger preterm labor. Alcohol may result in fetal alcohol syndrome, characterized by facial abnormalities, growth restriction, and neurological defects.	
Placental abruption	The placenta prematurely detaches, partially or completely, from the uterus. Risk factors: maternal hypertension, traumatic injury, cigarette smoking, and cocaine use. Partial detachment interferes with the functioning of the placenta, causing intrauterine growth restriction. Severe bleeding occurs with total detachment.	Provide supportive care in the left lateral position. Manage the patient's airway, ventilation, and oxygen supplementation (100%). Transport rapidly if there is severe bleeding or a risk of imminent preterm delivery. Start an IV access line and give NS for placental abruption.
Placenta previa	The placenta implants over or near the internal cervical opening. Implantation may be complete (covering the entire opening), partial, or marginal (to the edge of the cervical opening). Results in increased incidences of hemorrhage in the third trimester. Symptoms include painless bleeding after the 20th week of gestation.	Provide supportive care in the left lateral position. Manage the patient's airway, ventilation, and oxygen supplementation (100%). IV access line and NS. Transport rapidly if there is severe bleeding, high BP ≥160/110, seizures, or altered mental status. Provide ECG monitoring. Administer magnesium sulfate for preeclampsia/ eclampsia.
Pregnancy-induced hypertension/ Preeclampsia/ Eclampsia	Hypertension >140/90 associated with increased protein in the urine and edema (peripheral or generalized) or increase of ≥ 5 pounds of weight in one week after the 20th week of gestation. Severe preeclampsia is BP ≥ 160/110. Symptoms include headache, abdominal pain, and visual disturbances. May progress to eclampsia (seizures) and death.	

Complication	Characteristic	Prehospital Interventions
Cephalic (vertex) presentation	**Military**: Head straight, neck not flexed. **Brow**: Neck extended, brow presents first, can cause birth trauma, so episiotomy or cesarean section (C-section) is usually required. **Face**: Severely extended neck with face presentation, may prolong labor, increase swelling of the fetus, and cause neck trauma.	Provide supportive care. Manage the patient's airway, ventilation, and oxygen supplementation (100%). Transport rapidly.
Breech presentation	**Frank breech** (buttocks presentation with legs extended upward) is the most common, but **single- or double-footling breech** (incomplete breech) or **buttocks** presentation with legs flexed (complete breech) can also occur. Breech presentation is most common with placenta previa, hydramnios, fetal anomalies, and multiple gestations. Cord prolapse is more likely. Head trauma may occur because molding does not occur, and the head can become entrapped.	

PROLAPSE OF THE UMBILICAL CORD

A prolapse of the umbilical cord occurs when the umbilical cord precedes the fetus in the birth canal and becomes entrapped by the descending fetus. With an **occult cord prolapse**, the umbilical cord is beside or just ahead of the fetal head. With a **nuchal cord prolapse**, the cord tightly wraps about the fetal neck. About half of the time, prolapses occur in the second stage of labor and relate to premature delivery, multiple gestations, or other complications. As contractions occur and the head descends, pressure to the umbilical cord occludes the blood flow, causing hypoxia and bradycardia. The decrease in blood flow through the umbilical vessels can cause impaired gas exchange, and if pressure on the cord is not relieved, the fetus can suffer severe neurological damage or death.

Prehospital Interventions: Elevate the presenting part off the cord, pull the cord off of the fetus's neck if possible, elevate the mother's knees to the chest to relieve pressure on the cord, provide 100% oxygen, and transport rapidly.

HYPEREMESIS GRAVIDARUM (HG) AND RH INCOMPATIBILITY

About 60–80% of pregnant woman suffer from nausea and vomiting (N/V), especially during the first trimester, but only about 2% suffer **hyperemesis gravidarum** (HG). Symptoms of HG include severe (sometimes intractable) N/V, weight loss, and dehydration.

Prehospital Interventions: Provide intravenous fluids with 5% glucose in NS or Ringer's lactate; administer antiemetic drugs, including promethazine (Phenergan), prochlorperazine (Compazine), or chlorpromazine (Thorazine).

Rh incompatibility occurs if the mother is Rh-negative and the father is Rh-positive, putting their infant at risk for hemolytic disease of the newborn (HDN). The blood from an Rh-positive baby can mix with the Rh-negative blood of the mother, causing the mother's immune system to make antibodies to destroy the Rh factor. This immune response is called Rh sensitization and can occur during C-section or vaginal delivery, miscarriage, abortion, placental abruption, amniocentesis, chorionic villus sampling, ectopic pregnancy, toxemia, and trauma during pregnancy. Women who are Rh-negative with an Rh-positive mate receive the serum RhoGAM, containing anti-Rh (anti-D) immunoglobulin in order to agglutinate any fetal red blood cells that pass over into the mother's circulatory system and thus prevent the mother from forming antibodies against them that will attack the infant and sensitize her for future pregnancies.

MULTIPLE GESTATIONS

In vitro fertilization and ovulation-inducing drugs have increased the incidence of high-order **multiple gestations** over the past 30 years. The trend of delayed childbearing has led to an increase in twin/multiple gestations. Infants born from multiple gestations are more likely to be born prematurely and with low birth weights. The incidence of premature birth and low birth weight is proportional to the number of fetuses. There may be growth restriction/growth discordance, oligohydramnios, and restriction of movement of one or more fetuses. Approximately 50% of twins and 90% of triplets are born premature, compared to 10% of singletons. With this increase in prematurity and proportion of infants born with low birth weight, there are increased morbidities, such as cerebral palsy and intellectual disabilities. The risk for genetic disorders, such as neural tube defects and GI and cardiac abnormalities, is twice that of single gestations.

Gynecological Emergencies

FEMALE REPRODUCTIVE SYSTEM

The female reproductive system includes the ovaries, fallopian tubes, uterus, cervix, vagina, vulva, labia minora, labia majora, clitoris, and breasts. Functions include ovulation, fertilization, menstruation, pregnancy, and lactation. **Menarche** (onset of menses) is usually between 9 and 15, but it may occur in younger girls and should be considered as a possibility with younger girls. **Menopause** occurs at approximately age 50, usually following a period of about 10 years of irregular periods during which time the person may become pregnant. The normal menstrual cycle is 28 days, but it may be up to 45 days in adolescents. Assessment should include abdominal or vaginal pain, vaginal bleeding or discharge, fever, nausea and vomiting, and dizziness. Patients should have their privacy protected during an examination, and the EMS provider should communicate openly, asking for permission to touch the patient. The provider should consider the possibility of pregnancy or sexually transmitted infection (STI) with any abnormal condition.

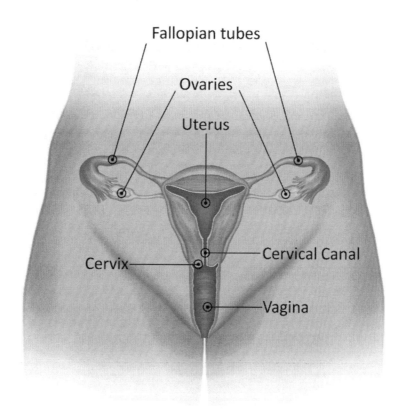

133

VAGINAL BLEEDING

Vaginal bleeding may indicate heavy menstrual bleeding (**menorrhagia**) or abnormal bleeding between cycles (**metrorrhagia**). Vaginal bleeding may also be an indication of an ectopic pregnancy or spontaneous abortion; in postmenopausal women, it may be a sign of endometrial cancer. Menorrhagia may result from hormonal imbalance, clotting disorders, uterine fibroids, and endometrial polyps. Metrorrhagia may result from infection, cancer, and cervical/endometrial polyps. Symptoms may include cramping and abdominal pain, depending on the cause. It's important to determine when the bleeding started and about how much blood has been lost (the number of sanitary pads that are saturated per hour, for example) as well as the presence or absence of pain. If the blood loss is excessive, the patient may exhibit signs of shock.

Prehospital Interventions: Use standard precautions, manage the patient's airway, ventilation, and oxygen as needed. Monitor vital signs. Position the patient flat for shock and provide IV access and fluids.

SEXUAL ASSAULT AND LEGAL ISSUES

The **crime scenes** associated with a **sexual assault** include the patient (body, injuries, clothing, and emotional response) and the place the assault occurred. A victim of sexual assault has the right to consent to or refuse each element of a sexual assault evaluation, although some states may mandate reporting of sexual assault to the authorities. The EMS provider should wear disposable gloves when handling clothing, and clothing should be handled gently so that evidence, such as strands of hair or other materials, is not lost in transfer. Documenting the assault should be done in detail with direct quotations. If the patient refuses transport, the best approach is to point out services that could benefit the patient, such as prophylaxis to prevent STIs and pregnancy. Patients are often frightened and confused, so pressuring them to protect others or trying to frighten them more by suggesting that they might be pregnant or develop an STI is a negative approach that may backfire.

Special Populations

INITIAL CARE OF THE NEWBORN

Dr. Virginia Apgar developed the **APGAR assessment** in 1952. APGAR stands for **a**ppearance, **p**ulse, **g**rimace, **a**ctivity, and **r**espiration. The APGAR is the first test given to a newborn. It is used as a quick evaluation of a newborn's physical condition to determine if any emergency medical care is needed, and it is administered 1 minute and 5 minutes after birth. The test is administered more than once because the baby's condition may change rapidly. It may be administered for a third time 10 minutes after birth if needed. The baby is rated on the five subscales, and scores are added together. A total score of ≥7 is a sign of good health.

Sign	0	1	2
Appearance (skin color)	Cyanotic or pallor over entire body	Acrocyanosis	Pink
Pulse (heart rate)	Absent	<100 bpm	>100 bpm
Grimace (reflex irritability)	Unresponsive	Grimace	Infant sneezes, coughs, and recoils
Activity (muscle tone)	Absent	Flexed limbs	Infant moves freely
Respiration (breathing rate and effort)	Absent	Slow, irregular; weak cry	Vigorous cry

> **Review Video: Newborn APGAR Score**
> Visit mometrix.com/academy and enter code: 253451

ROUTINE CARE OF THE NEWBORN

Infants have poor temperature regulation ability, particularly preterm infants who lack brown fat, which is one of the body's tools to regulate body temperature, so **providing warmth** is critical as a component of resuscitation. An infant who is just seconds old and wet will need aggressive measures to keep him or her warm while any resuscitation efforts are being initiated. Infants lose heat through their heads, so one of the first steps should be to place a hat on the head or cover the head in some way. The infant should be vigorously dried with warmed blankets. Often, this stimulation, drying and warming, is all that is needed to establish a regular respiration pattern in the neonate. Preterm infants weighing <1500 grams should be placed in a plastic bag (made specifically for this purpose), if available, up to the height of the shoulders to prevent cold shock. A term infant with no distress can be placed on the mother's chest and covered with a warm blanket.

ABCs of Resuscitation of the Neonate

The **ABCs of resuscitation** should begin immediately after delivery with assisted ventilation begun within 60 seconds if required.

- **Airway:** An airway should be established as the very first thing tended to; if there is no airway, air cannot be moved during resuscitation attempts. This step includes using a bulb syringe to clear the mouth, then the nose of secretions and properly positioning the infant's head in the sniffing position.
- **Breathing**: This step involves initiating breathing after the airway has been established; this can be done with stimulation, supplemental oxygen, or through artificial ventilation if there is apnea, gasping, or heart rate below 100 bpm. Attach pulse oximeter, consider cardiac monitor, and give PPV at 40-60 breaths per minute.
- **Circulation**: Start compressions if heart rate is <60 bpm after 30 seconds of PPV with chest movement. Check HR every 60 seconds. Compress one-third of the anterior-posterior diameter of the chest, using two thumbs or two fingers. Give 3 compressions to 1 breath every 2 seconds (90 compressions to 30 ventilations per minute). Increase oxygen to 100% during compressions. If the HR remains <60 bpm after 60 seconds of CPR, administer epinephrine by IV or ET. Volume expanders (isotonic crystalloid at 10 mL/kg) can be given IV if the neonate is hypovolemic.

Establishing an Airway

To establish an airway, the infant is placed supine with the head slightly extended in the sniffing position. A small neck roll may be placed under the shoulders to maintain this position in a very small premature infant. Once the proper position is established, the mouth and nose are suctioned (suction the mouth first to prevent reflex inspiration of secretions when the nose is suctioned) with a bulb syringe or catheter if necessary. The infant's head can be turned momentarily to the side to allow secretions to pool in the cheek where they can be more easily suctioned and removed to establish the airway. Stimulating the newborn is often all that is needed to initiate spontaneous respirations. This tactile stimulation can be accomplished by gently rubbing the back or trunk of the infant. Another technique that is used to provide stimulation is flicking or rubbing the soles of the feet. Slapping neonates as stimulation is no longer practiced and should NOT be used.

Managing Airway and Ventilation

Airway management is based on the severity of respiratory distress:

- **Blow-by oxygen**: Provide if the newborn is cyanotic and heart rate is >100 bpm and respiratory effort is adequate. Provide warm oxygen at 5 L/min. with a direct flow on the face. Avoid oral airways.
- **Bag-valve mask (BVM)**: Provide if the newborn is apneic, the heart rate <100, and/or there is inadequate respiratory effort. Use an appropriate size and avoid excess pressure, which may cause pneumothorax, although initial ventilation requires higher pressure to expand the lungs. Disable the pop-off valve.
- **Intubation**: Provide if other measures are ineffective and the heart rate is <60. Use a straight-blade laryngoscope size #1 for full term and size #0 for preterm with ETT 2.5-4.0 mm, depending on the weight of newborn. Confirm placement through visualization, auscultation (lateral, superior chest wall, epigastric region), improvement in respirations, ETCO$_2$ detector, and pulse oximetry. Secure the ETT. Provide PEEP as indicated at 5 cmH$_2$O. Gastric decompression may be necessary if the abdomen is distended. Provide CPR as needed.

GROWTH AND DEVELOPMENT OF PEDIATRIC PATIENTS

Normal growth and development by age, in the first two years of life, is as follows:

- **0–2 months**: Sleeps up to 16 hours per day but should rouse easily. Cries for a reason; persistent crying may indicate illness. Limited head control. Gazes at faces.
- **2–6 months**: Smiles voluntarily and makes eye contact, uses both hands, begins to hold his or her head up, rolls over, and sleeps through the night.
- **6–12 months**: Sits, crawls, has pincer grasp, mouths objects (increasing risk of poisoning and aspiration), babbles, and speaks first words by 12 months. Exhibits separation anxiety from parents.
- **12–18 months**: Begins to walk; imitates others; knows body parts and 4-6 words; lacks molars for grinding food, increasing the risk of aspiration; and has increased mobility.
- **18–24 months**: Begins to run and climb, knows 100 words (24 months), clings to parents, attaches to special objects, labels objects, and begins to understand cause and effect.
- **2–5 years**: Walks, runs, throws, catches, is toilet trained, has magical thinking and irrational fears, learns acceptable behavior, has temper tantrums, and develops modesty.
- **6–12 years**: Loses baby teeth; thinks logically; becomes self-conscious; understands the finality of death; attaches importance to school, popularity, and peers.
- **12–20 years**: Puberty begins, reasons (imperfectly), is self-conscious, seeks independence and peer approval, and takes risks.

PEDIATRIC CONSIDERATIONS

Pediatric patients have the following physiologic considerations:

- Proportionately greater body surface area to body mass ratio, so they are at greater risk of fluid and heat loss, burns, and absorption of toxins
- Higher respiratory rates and heart rates than adults, resulting in higher oxygen demand
- Immature blood/brain barrier, resulting in more neurological symptoms
- Immature immune system, resulting in a higher risk of infection
- Narrower and shorter airway and smaller jaw, so the tongue may easily obstruct the airway
- Soft tracheal cartilage that increases the risk of airway collapse, and a large epiglottis
- More pliable ribs, which provide less protection for abdominal organs, which are more forward
- Liver and spleen that are proportionately larger and at risk of injury
- Bones that are softer with open growth plates (an open growth plate injury can impair growth)
- Less protection for the brain and spinal cord (increasing the risk of injury) and less subarachnoid space
- Cerebral blood flow needs twice that of adults, increasing the risk of hypoxia
- Limited glucose stores and risk of hypothermia (especially in the first month)
- Anterior fontanel that closes by 12 months and posterior fontanel that closes by 3-4 months

PEDIATRIC ASSESSMENT

The pediatric assessment should include the following:

- **Pediatric assessment triangle**:
  - *Appearance* (abnormal tone, decreased interactivity, decreased consolability, abnormal look/gaze, and abnormal speech or cry)
  - *Work of breathing* (abnormal sounds [wheezing, stridor], position, retractions [sternum], flaring [nostrils], and apnea/gasping)
  - *Circulation* (pallor, mottling, and cyanosis)
- **Assess airway, breathing, and circulation (heart rate/pulse)**: Place in the shock position and provide a warming blanket for signs of shock.
- **Ventilation/oxygenation**: Administer oxygen and assist with ventilation if it is abnormal.
- **Determine the patient's level of consciousness**: Use the alert, voice, pain, unresponsive (AVPU) assessment. Note movement of the extremities and whether the pupils are normal, dilated, constricted, reactive, or fixed.
- **Prevent hypothermia**: Cover with a warming blanket, cover the head, and avoid unnecessary exposure of the skin.
- **Obtain the medical history from the caregiver/parent**: Include the type and duration of symptoms, fever, level of activity, recent foods/fluids, medications, medication allergies, past or chronic illnesses, and events leading to the current problem.
- **Head-to-toe physical examination**: Note any bruising, swelling, drainage, loose teeth, unusual odors, bleeding, rashes, deformities, and pain on movement.

PEDIATRIC SEIZURES

Febrile seizure is a generalized seizure associated with fever, usually >38.8 °C (101.8 °F) from any type of infection (upper respiratory, urinary tract) but without intracranial infection or other cause, occurring between 6 months and 5 years of age. Seizures usually last <15 minutes and are without subsequent neurological deficit.

Prehospital Interventions: Provide fever control (acetaminophen OR ibuprofen) and a tepid-water bath.

Other types of seizures may result from pathology, such as meningitis, cerebral edema, brain trauma, or brain tumors, but most seizures in children >3 are related to idiopathic epilepsy, which predisposes the child to recurrent seizures, usually of the same type. Seizures are characterized as focal (localized), focal with rapid generalization (spreading), and generalized (widespread). In most children, seizures become generalized with loss of consciousness. Seizure disorders with onset younger than 4 years of age usually cause more neurological damage than those with onset at older than 4 years of age.

Prehospital Interventions: Place the patient on the floor or on a safe surface, loosen clothes, and protect him or her from injury during seizure. Afterward, place the patient in the recovery position, monitor the airway/ventilation, and provide oxygen supplementation (the patient may need assisted ventilation if he or she is cyanotic), and suction if needed.

BRIEF, RESOLVED, UNEXPLAINED EVENT AND SUDDEN INFANT DEATH SYNDROME

Brief, resolved, unexplained event (BRUE) refers to a group of alarming symptoms that can occur in infants. They involve a sudden appearance of apnea, altered responsiveness, and change in color or muscle tone. The event lasts <1 minute in an infant <1 year of age, in which there is no underlying cause, and there is a quick spontaneous return to their baseline state of health. With **sudden infant death syndrome (SIDS)**, which is almost always related to respiratory arrest, the child cannot be resuscitated. There are numerous proposed causes for SIDS, so a careful history, including familial history of SIDS, and physical examination or postmortem examination can provide important information, such as indications of child abuse or metabolic/infectious disorders.

Prehospital Interventions: Continue resuscitative efforts (airway, ventilation, oxygen supplementation, and compressions as indicated) and stabilize the infant if possible. The child with BRUE should be hospitalized for observation, further studies, and apnea monitoring because these children are at increased risk for SIDS. For SIDS patients, the EMS provider should provide support and information to the family. The protocol for reporting SIDS varies by state, but it usually involves notifying the coroner's office.

GERIATRIC CONSIDERATIONS

Geriatric patients have the following special considerations and characteristics:

- Decreased sensory input (hearing, vision, touch, pain), impaired depth perception and night vision, and decreased ability to differentiate colors
- Hypertension, increasing the risk of heart attack and stroke
- Decreased breathing capacity and decreased cough, increasing the risk of infection
- Difficulty chewing and swallowing, digestive problems, and reflux when lying flat, which increases the risk of aspiration
- Short-term memory deficit and slower reflexes
- Decreased bone density, increasing the risk of breaks; loss of muscle tone
- Increased risk of infection and less obvious symptoms of infection
- Arthritis in the neck, interfering with airway assessment
- Dentures that can obstruct the airway (leave them in place if possible, during ventilation)
- Skin that is fragile and tears easily
- Irregular pulse from underlying heart problems
- Dementia (incidence increases with age), making history taking and treatment difficult
- Atypical symptoms for illnesses, even if severely ill
- Multiple comorbidities and multiple medications
- Shock with BP greater than 100

ADDITIONAL PATIENT POPULATIONS WITH SPECIAL CHALLENGES

HOMELESS/INDIGENT

These patients often are without medical care, increasing the risk of disease, and they may lack insurance. They are more likely to have mental health and substance abuse problems.

Prehospital considerations: Know who will treat indigent patients and what resources are available in the community.

BARIATRIC

These patients have increased risk of chronic disease. Patients pose handling/moving problems and require special bariatric equipment and multiple personnel to assist. Patients often have trouble breathing and must have their head elevated.

Prehospital considerations: Recognize the need for bariatric equipment and know how/where to obtain it. Notify the receiving facility. Use properly sized equipment, such as BP cuffs.

TECHNOLOGY/DEVICE-ASSISTED

These patients may have a wide range of issues including ventilators, apnea monitors, vascular devices, dialysis shunts, colostomies, ileostomies, and feeding tubes. Patients may have special needs regarding care and transport.

Prehospital considerations: Ask about the patient's equipment and needs. Avoid disturbing/damaging the devices if possible.

EMS Operations

Overview of EMS Operations

APPARATUS AND EQUIPMENT READINESS

The EMS provider should ensure that the ambulance is ready for use at all times and that the tires are properly inflated, the gas tank is full, warning devices are working, and engine fluid levels are appropriate. All necessary safety equipment, such as PPE (masks, gowns, gloves, and goggles or face guards) and safety devices (safety vests, road flares, and signs) as well as seat belts and harnesses, should be available and in proper working condition. All equipment in the cab, the compartments, and the rear of the ambulance should be in the proper place, labeled, and secured to prevent shifting during transportation. High-risk situations include going through intersections, inclement weather (especially with poor visibility), careless drivers, highway access, unpaved roads, and driver distractions (conversation, eating, drinking, mobile devices, music, GPS devices, and fatigue). During transportation, all personnel as well as patients should be properly secured with safety equipment.

SCENE-OF-INCIDENT SAFETY CONSIDERATIONS

The EMS provider must do a 360° **assessment of the scene of incident** on arrival and determine safety considerations. The provider should make note of any gunshots heard, downed power lines, buildings in a state of collapse, leaking fuels/fluids, fire, smoke, broken glass, and other hazards. EMS personnel may need to wait until the site is safe to proceed. The EMS provider should assess the mechanism of injury (accidents) and the need for appropriate PPE (gloves, gown, mask, face guard) and must keep the patient informed of all actions and prevent harm or further injury. The ambulance should be parked off of the roadway if possible or parked at a 45° angle (front wheels out) to shield the work area, making sure not to block access for other emergency vehicles. Parking uphill is safer than downhill, and upwind is safer than downwind. If flares are used to warn other drivers, they should extend at least 300 feet from a collision. Yellow warning lights at the scene are the safest, but excessive lighting may blind other drivers at night.

ENVIRONMENTAL RISK FACTORS

When assessing a patient, it's important to consider that **environmental factors** may place the patient at an increased risk for harm or may be a factor in disease. There are a number of different types of environmental factors to consider.

Factors	Examples	Effects
Toxic chemicals	Lead, arsenic, muriatic acid, sulfuric acid, ammonia, lime	May result in poisoning (lead, arsenic) or burns (acids, ammonia, lime) through direct exposure or inhalation
Physical objects	Guns, cars, knives, equipment	Accidents, gunshot wounds, stabbings, various injuries (blunt and penetrating)
Biological organisms	Bacteria, fungi, viruses	Infections
Temperature variations	Heat, cold	Burns, dehydration, heat stroke, hyperthermia, hypothermia, frostbite
Ambient noise	Sirens, loud music, traffic noise, work-related noise	Hearing loss/deafness, increased anxiety
Psychosocial	Increased stress	Anxiety, hypertension, suicidal ideation

141

RESCUES IN CONFINED SPACES

A confined space is one in which access is limited and the space is surrounded by walls or structures that are not suitable for habitation. A **confined space** may occur in a building (such as with a collapse), a silo, a motor vehicle (such as a large vehicle involved in a crash), a cistern or septic tank, or a well. A confined space may pose a risk to the patient and EMS personnel because of difficulty moving about and accessing the patient as well as decreased ventilation that may result in the buildup of toxic gases and/or a lack of oxygen. Before entering a confined space, the EMS provider should test the atmosphere and use the correct breathing equipment. This is especially important if the patient is nonresponsive, which is often an indication of poor air quality. The provider should also carefully assess his or her ability to access the patient and the best means of doing so.

TRANSFERRING A PATIENT FROM THE SCENE TO AN AMBULANCE

Different types of **stretchers** and **transfer equipment** may be used for prehospital transfer, including the following:

- **Wheeled**: Stretcher that can be lowered and raised with a wheeled base allowing it to slide into the ambulance.
- **Scoop**: Two- to four-piece stretcher that can be connected and placed under a patient.
- **Transfer sheet**: A heavy plastic sheet can be used with patients up to 800 lb to facilitate transfer.
- **Flexible stretcher**: Lightweight flexible (plastic, rubberized canvas) stretcher with webbing handles on both sides. Can be used to transfer patients around corners and up and down stairs where a wheeled stretcher cannot be used.
- **Stair chair**: Safety chair that can be used to transfer patients in tight spaces and up and down stairs.
- **Folding stretcher**: A stretcher made of lightweight materials that allows folding for compact storage in an ambulance.
- **Basket stretcher** (Stokes basket): Used primarily for rescues in the wilderness or from cliffs.

PATIENT POSITIONING

Patient positioning should be according to the possible or probable injury, with safety restraints always securing the patient to the gurney and the gurney to the vehicle.

- **Left-side-lying:** Pregnant patients should be placed in this position to increase circulation to the placenta, and unconscious patients should be placed in this position to prevent aspiration and choking if there is no indication of a spinal injury.
- **Supine** (flat on the back): Patient has a suspected pelvic fracture or neck injury (also requires a cervical collar).
- **Supine** (feet elevated above the heart): This is the position for patients in shock to increase circulation to the heart and brain as the BP falls.
- **Trendelenburg** (the entire stretcher is tilted so that the head is below the feet): Position for patients with a suspected spinal cord injury.
- **Semi-Fowler's** (30-45° position): For patients with chest pain, stroke, and/or shortness of breath and no indication of a spinal cord injury.
- **Fowler's** (upright, 90° position): For patients with severe shortness of breath.

BACKBOARDS AND CERVICAL COLLARS

Backboards were originally designed to transfer patients. However, **backboards and cervical collars** have been routinely used for EMS rescues for many years without evidence-based studies supporting their use. The premise was that stabilizing the spine and neck would prevent further injury in case a spinal injury had occurred, but spinal injuries are relatively rare, and some studies indicate that these devices do not provide any protection and, in fact, may cause damage. Additionally, cervical collars restrict the airway by 20% or more and may worsen injuries if not properly sized for the patient. Because of these findings, some EMS no longer routinely use backboards but use a vacuum mattress in a scoop basket instead. The American Association of Neurological Surgeons/Congress of Neurological Surgeons (AANS/CNS) 2013 guidelines advise that spinal immobilization using a backboard be reserved for known or suspected spinal cord injury without penetrating injury, although the use of the cervical collar is still recommended until the cervical spine is assessed for injury. Short backboards may be used to support a patient's back in a sitting position.

EMERGENCY MOVES

Emergency moves may be needed if the patient and/or EMS provider is in immediate danger from fire, explosives, or other hazards; if the patient requires life-saving treatment, such as cardiopulmonary resuscitation (CPR); or if the patient is in water, such as a pond or lake. **Emergency moves** include the following:

- **Blanket drag**: Logroll the patient onto a blanket, wrap the patient in the blanket, grasp the blanket near the patient's head while in a squatting position with your back straight, and drag. If there are two rescuers, the other should be positioned at the patient's feet and should be pushing.
- **Clothing drag**: Squat down by the patient's head, securely grasp the clothing near the patient's neck or shoulders (avoid grasping by a T-shirt), and drag the patient.
- **Arm drag**: Squat down by the patient's head. Fold the patient's arms across his or her chest. Grasp the patient under the arms, wrapping your arms about the torso and grasping the patient's wrists to stabilize his or her arms. Drag the patient.

Urgent moves, such as with altered mental status, shock, or breathing difficulties, should also be done as quickly as possible.

Emergency moves can be carried out by one rescuer if no other assistance is available, as follows:

- **Firefighter's drag**: Tie the patient's wrists together with any available material. Straddle the patient and pull the patient's arms over your neck and then crawl forward, dragging him or her beneath you.

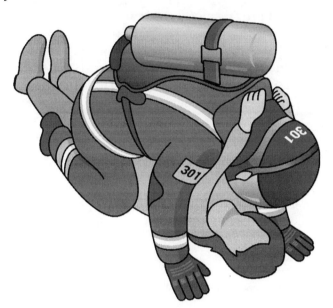

- **Firefighter's carry**: Grasp the patient's knees and pull them together and up. Stand on the patient's feet and reach out and grab one of the patient's arms with one hand. Pull the patient upright, and, as the patient elevates, place your other hand between the patient's legs. Place the patient's arm behind your neck and continue to pull the patient and lift until he or she is draped across your upper back with the arm hanging free. Then grasp the patient's arm that is hanging with the hand that is between the legs to secure the patient.

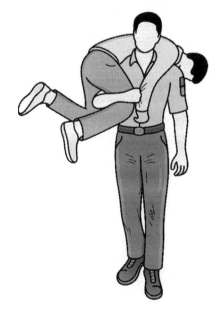

DRIVING SAFETY

The **ambulance driver** should stop briefly or slow significantly at intersections because other drivers may not hear or may ignore sirens. The driver should keep the brake covered with the left foot for fast braking and avoid excessive speeds because of the increased risk of accidents, especially on curves. The speed should be adjusted for road and weather conditions and should not be influenced by use of the siren (siren syndrome). Snow and ice should be cleared from the ambulance before driving it. At least one vehicle length should separate the ambulance from other vehicles for every 10 mph of speed. A spotter should always be used when backing up the ambulance because of poor visibility. All personnel in the ambulance should be seated and secured with seat belts or safety harnesses before the ambulance moves. Studies have shown that CPR is most effective if done from a sitting position in an ambulance rather than standing, despite common practice. Patients and gurneys should also be secured.

LIGHTS AND SIRENS

Lights and sirens should be used together, and they are indicated when going to a scene and when transporting a patient in a serious emergent situation. There are four types of warning lights used on emergency vehicles such as ambulances: rotating lights (resulting in a flashing sensation), fixed flashes (usually red or blue), strobe lights, and LED lights. Red (the most common) and blue lights are generally used to indicate emergency vehicles and can be used to obtain the right-of-way or to block the right-of-way. These colors may be interchangeable, although in some states the color blue is restricted to law enforcement vehicles. Amber lights are warning lights and can be used by all vehicles, but they do not require others to stop. Some emergency vehicle lights change to amber when the vehicle is parked. Green lights are sometimes used to indicate a mobile incident command post, but in some states, green lights may also indicate private security vehicles or volunteer firefighters.

Incident Management

FEMA IS-700.A NIMS

FEMA IS-700.A outlines the **National Incident Management System (NIMS)**, which, under the direction of the **Federal Emergency Management Agency (FEMA)**, an agency of the U.S. Department of Homeland Security, provides the foundation for collaboration among different governmental and nongovernmental agencies, jurisdictions, and specialties/disciplines in handling large-scale incidents that threaten life, property, and/or the environment. Components of FEMA IS-700.A include the following:

- **Preparedness**: Focuses on planning, procedures and protocols, training and exercises, personnel qualifications/certification, and equipment certification, and it includes the National Response Framework, which establishes protocols and ensures that local jurisdictions retain control while still using a unified approach.
- **Communications and information management**: Systems must be interoperable, reliable, portable, scalable, resilient, and redundant.
- **Resource management**: This includes personnel, equipment, supplies, and facilities, which must be inventoried and categorized using a standardized approach.
- **Command and management**: This includes the Incident Command System (this standardized approach outlines the responsibilities of the incident commander, area command, command staff, and general staff), multiagency coordination systems, and public information.
- **Management and maintenance**: The National Integration Center (NIC) is responsible for NIMS management.
- **Flexibility**: Components are scalable and adaptable to all types of incidents.
- **Standardization**: The NIC develops standards in cooperation with standards development organizations.

ICS-100.B

ICS-100.B, the **Incident Command System** course, meets NIMS requirements for operational personnel and outlines a standardized approach to incident management. ICS is used for any type of major event, planned or otherwise, and large- or small-scale incidents, including natural (disasters), technological (hazmat release), and human-caused (civil disturbance) hazards. ICS outlines the chain of command; the incident commander is in control and orders go through supervisors. Every incident requires an incident action plan, resource management, and processes for reimbursement. The incident commander establishes an incident command post and staging areas (gathering places) as well a base (coordination area for logistic and administrative functions), camps (for sleeping, eating, and sanitary services), helibases, and helispots. Primary features of ICS include common terminology, establishment/transfer of command, chain of command/unity of command, management of objects, incident action planning, modular organization, manageable span of control, comprehensive resource management, incident facilities and locations, integrated communications, information and intelligence management, accountability, and dispatch/deployment.

CHAIN OF COMMAND, UNITY OF COMMAND AND UNIFIED COMMAND

Each organization must establish the **chain of command** for its incident command system. Although these may vary somewhat, an incident commander is ultimately in charge with individuals assigned as incident managers in different areas, such as triage, treatment, transport, security, and liaison.

Unity of command means that each incident commander should have control over personnel assigned to his or her area, and each individual within the chain of command should have a clear understanding of whom to report to at the scene so that communication is efficient and timely.

Unified command means that when multiple agencies are involved from multiple jurisdictions, the chain of command that has been established is recognized and respected even though each agency retains its own authority and accountability and is responsible for carrying out its own duties. A unified command system prevents duplication of effort as well as neglect of important functions.

INCIDENT ACTION PLAN

The purpose of the **incident action plan** is to outline control objectives, resources, and strategies for dealing with an incident. Incident action plans should be updated frequently. Incident action plans may be designed for various types of incidents (terrorist attack, disease outbreak, hurricane) and modified as needed and should include the following:

- Goals and objectives, including expected outcomes
- Strategies and tactics for responding and accomplishing the goals and objectives
- An outline of the chain of command for the incident command system, including the span of control (the number of people reporting to an individual)
- Tasks assigned to each level in the chain of command
- Safety/Health plan for responders to prevent injury/illness and to treat victims as needed
- Communications plan outlining how information will be exchanged, including alternative methods of command if, for example, cell phone towers are out of commission
- Logistics plan regarding the acquisition and use of resources, such as supplies, personnel, and equipment
- Maps and demographic information

INCIDENT COMMANDER

When a multiple-casualty or mass-casualty event occurs, the first lead emergency medical responder on the scene generally assumes the role of **incident commander**, carries out a rapid assessment of the scene, and calls for additional resources as indicated while another medical responder begins triage. The incident commander should begin to establish a command center in an area that is safe and out of the way of emergency vehicles while awaiting assistance. This first incident commander will relinquish the role when the staffed and/or assigned incident commander arrives to take command and should then report to the person who is assuming the role of staging officer. The incident commander's duties include establishing command, assessing needs, developing a plan, coordinating all activities, delegating responsibilities, ensuring the safety of all personnel and patients, liaising with other agencies, and communicating information.

TRIAGE

PRIMARY TRIAGE AND RESOURCE MANAGEMENT

Primary triage is a rapid method (30–60 seconds) of prioritizing patients based on the severity of their condition, and it is carried out at the scene of multiple-casualty incidents. All patients are triaged and tagged according to the following international color-coding priority (P) guidelines on the foot or wrist (not on the clothing):

- **P1—Red**: Immediate care is needed for urgent systemic life-threatening conditions, such as airway/breathing problems, severe bleeding, severe burns (especially with breathing problems), decreased mental status, shock, and severe medical problems, or a Glasgow Coma Scale score of ≤13.

- **P2—Yellow**: Delayed care, patient is able to wait 45–60 minutes for treatment. Conditions include burns (without breathing problems), multiple bone/joint injuries, back and/or spinal cord injuries (unless the patient is in respiratory distress).
- **P3—Green**: Hold, patient is able to wait hours for treatment of minor injuries.
- **P4—Black**: Patient is deceased.

Resource management involves identifying a triage officer, who remains at the scene during the event and identifying the need for additional personnel and equipment and providing those to the patients with the highest priority.

SECONDARY TRIAGE/RE-TRIAGE

During a mass-casualty incident, triage is done quickly, and patients may be scattered over a wide area with many patients being red-tagged for emergency care. Patients coded black are left in place, but those with other-color tags should be moved and segregated in separate sections of a holding area to await treatment and/or transport. The patients should be **re-triaged** as they are moved into the holding area to determine if the tagging color is still appropriate. Additionally, **secondary triage** may be carried out in the separate sections, especially if some must be airlifted, to determine which patients have the best chance of survival and should receive priority for transfer and treatment. Secondary triage may also help to determine which trauma center (based on location or level of care) or hospital is most appropriate for the patient considering the patient's condition, transport time, and the surge capacity of the healthcare institutions.

CDC GUIDELINES FOR FIELD TRIAGE OF INJURED PATIENTS

The CDC's guidelines for field triage of injured patients is a four-step algorithm that is used to identify the most seriously ill patients and transport them to an appropriate treatment center.

Step	Assess	Findings requiring priority treatment	Plan
1	Vital signs/ Level of consciousness	Glasgow Coma Scale score of ≤13, systolic BP <90 mm Hg, respiratory rate <10 or >29 per minute (<20 in an infant <1 year), or need of ventilatory support.	Highest level trauma center
2	Anatomy of injury	Penetrating injuries, flail chest, two or more long-bone fractures, crushed/mangled/pulseless extremity, amputations, pelvic fractures, open/depressed skull fracture, or paralysis.	Highest level trauma center
3	Mechanism of injury/High-energy impact	Falls—adults >20 feet and children >10 feet or 2–3 times their height. High-risk auto crash with intrusions, partial or complete ejection, or there is a death in the same passenger compartment. Auto vs. pedestrian/bicycle with victim thrown, run over, or sustaining a significant impact. Motorcycle crash >20 mph.	Trauma center
4	Special patient/ system considerations	Older adults, children, pregnancy >30 weeks, burns, patients on anticoagulants or with bleeding disorders (based on the EMS provider's best judgment).	Trauma center/ hospital

START METHOD OF TRIAGE

With the START method of triage, the EMS provider starts triage with the first victim encountered, tags the patient, and then moves to the next patient, assessing in order: (1) respirations, (2) perfusion, and (3) mental status (RPM) and using the standard red-yellow-green-black color-coding system. Walking wounded are tagged as green.

Respirations	Present	Red tag if >30 Continue to perfusion assessment if <30
	Not present—position the airway	Red tag if respirations recur or black tag (death) if none
Perfusion	Radial pulse absent or capillary refill of greater than 2 seconds	Control bleeding and red tag
	Radial pulse present and capillary refill time of less than 2 seconds	Continue to mental status assessment
Mental status	Cannot follow simple directions	Red tag
	Can follow simple directions	Yellow tag

JUMPSTART METHOD OF TRIAGE FOR PEDIATRIC PATIENTS

JumpSTART is a pediatric triage method developed only for use in multiple-casualty incidents.

Able to walk	No	Continue to breathing assessment.
	Yes	Green tag. Carry out secondary triage.
Breathing	No	Step 1: Position upper airway and red tag if breathing. Step 2: Give five rescue breaths and red tag if breathing. Black tag if breathing does not recur.
	Yes	Respiratory rate <15 or >45, red tag. Respiratory rate 15 to 45, continue to pulse assessment.
Palpable pulse	No	Red tag.
	Yes	Continue to AVPU assessment.
Alert, voice, pain, unresponsive (AVPU) assessment	Inappropriate pain, posturing, or unresponsive	Red tag.
	A, V, or P is appropriate	Yellow tag.

AIR MEDICAL TRANSPORT

Air medical transport is indicated when the patient is in need of a high level of care that may be available on an aircraft but not an ambulance, when the patient's condition and need for treatment are time critical, when the patient is located in a remote area where access by ambulance is difficult or would be delayed (helicopter), or when local medical services have exceeded their capacity. Helipads are often available at large hospitals, so the patient can be treated immediately after arrival. Some disadvantages include inclement weather (which may interfere with flight plans) as well as altitude and airspeed limitations. Depending on the aircraft, the cabin size may be inadequate for the patient, personnel, and equipment. Difficult terrain, such as forested or hilly areas may not provide an adequate landing site. Cost is the biggest difference between ground and air transport with air transport often costing tens of thousands of dollars with only part, or in some cases none, of the costs being covered by insurance.

Mometrix

HELICOPTERS

Helicopters have the advantage over fixed-wing aircraft of being able to load a patient at or near the scene rather than having to transport the patient by ambulance to an airport. A paved surface is not necessary for a helicopter landing site, but level grassy or paved sites are preferred, ideally with 100 × 100 feet of clear space, but a minimum area of 60 × 60 feet may be used. Additionally, the area should be free of debris that may be disrupted by the rotor blades and should be clear of structures that may interfere with the aircraft, such as power poles, tall trees, power lines, cables, and antennas. A rotor aircraft does not require that people approach in a crouching position, but people should avoid holding anything over their heads and should generally approach from the front of the aircraft and avoid the rear of the aircraft and the rear rotors.

SAFETY ISSUES DURING AIR TRANSPORT

The pilot in command (PIC) of rotorcraft and fixed-wing aircraft is responsible for the **safety** of the aircraft, crew, emergency medical personnel, and the patient. As with all takeoffs and landings, medical staff and crew must be seated and secured by seat belts. Helmets should be in place and secure. Patients who are violent, confused, or combative should be physically restrained for transport and may also require chemical restraints to ensure their own personal safety as well as the safety of the medical and flight crew. Patients should be offloaded ONLY when a crew member signals the receiving medical personnel to approach the aircraft. With high-altitude fixed-wing air transports, cabins are pressurized but only to the equivalent of 6000–8000 feet, not to sea level. Rotorcraft are usually used to transfer a patient from the scene of an incident to a primary care facility or from the primary care facility to another type of facility, whereas a fixed-wing aircraft is usually used from one facility to another over longer distances.

COMMUNICATION ISSUES

A **communication specialist** should coordinate all air medical services, including communications within an agency and between agencies regarding all aspects of transport. The communication specialist should have radio communication skills and knowledge of medical terminology, including knowledge of how to obtain information about a patient, navigation, map usage, customer service, weather, aircraft emergencies, as well as **Federal Aviation Administration (FAA)** and **Federal Communications Commission (FCC)** regulations that relate to air medical transport. The communication specialist should be familiar with radio frequencies used by EMS. The dispatcher determines whether an aircraft should take off. The communication center may be located in a medical facility, airport, or other space, but it should be free of distractions and have emergency backup electrical power. All air medical transport team members should have knowledge of the radio communication system. Some systems include radio or radio-phone communication, and some systems require the team members to carry pagers, such as two-way satellite pagers. All incoming and outgoing communication should be recorded.

STATE AND FEDERAL REGULATIONS

State **statutes** require that aircraft used for air ambulance service must be licensed to provide that service, and the service must ensure that all required medical equipment is available. Although statutes may vary slightly from one state to another, most require that the service be able to provide basic and advanced life support and should provide patients with a description of services and costs. Additionally, the aircraft and crew must comply with FAA regulations and carry insurance to cover injuries that may occur in transport. The FAA carries out periodic inspections of aircraft and issues resource documents regarding safety and operations. Federal regulations establish weather guidelines for safe flying. The **U.S. Department of Transportation** provides guidelines regarding standards of care. The **Commission on Accreditation of Medical Transport**

Systems establishes voluntary accreditation standards, but air medical services associated with hospitals must meet hospital accreditation standards, typically those of the Joint Commission.

SAFE EXTRICATION FROM A MOTOR VEHICLE (CAR, TRUCK)
SCENE MANAGEMENT

Scene management at the site of an accident that requires vehicle extrication incudes initial evaluation of any hazards at the site (360° evaluation), such as oncoming traffic, fallen wires, spilled fuel, and fire/explosion risk or presence. The scene must be secured (45° parking, police security, flares, and cones) and the EMS provider should don protective equipment as necessary and access the patient to provide life-saving care. The patient must be disentangled from the motor vehicle as much as can be done safely. The patient is prepared for extrication (such as by applying pressure to bleeding sites and placing a cervical collar), removed from the vehicle, and then prepared for ground or air transport and provided emergent treatment. For extrications in difficult terrain, assess the following:

- **Terrain**: Forests, desert, cliff, water, snow
- **Obstacles**: Trees, rocks, light, unavailability of landing sites
- **Methods to be used**: Helicopter extrication, overland carry, or other type of extrication
- **Alternative solutions**: Abort, contact search and rescue
- **Safety issues**: Review all safety concerns

INITIAL ACTIONS

For **vehicle extrication**, the vehicle must be stabilized before the EMS personnel attempt to enter the vehicle or administer aid to the patient, especially if the vehicle may slide or is on its side and the personnel must access the vehicle from the top because the vehicle may shift and further endanger the patient as well as EMS personnel. EMS personnel can access the vehicle through a window, breaking it if necessary, or a door if one is operable (the patient may be able to assist in opening a window or door). EMS personnel should carry an airway (in case the patient requires ventilation), dressings (to apply pressure if the patient is bleeding), and a rigid cervical collar (to protect against spinal injury or further spinal damage) and should do rapid triage on access to the patient. Oxygen is usually not administered until after the patient is extracted because of the danger of fire, especially if the patient is saturated with fuel, and CPR is not done until the patient is in the supine position on a solid surface. If patients are apneic and pulseless, they must be removed as quickly as possible even with only manual protection of the spine being provided.

EXTRICATION PROCESS

For vehicle extrication, once EMS personnel have gained access to the motor vehicle, they should unlock its doors, if possible, to allow others to more easily gain access. The EMS personnel should ensure that the engine is turned off, the parking brake is set, and the transmission is set to park. If possible, an emergency response person should disconnect the battery to decrease the risk of fire and explosion. If the patient can be removed, a short backboard should be applied before moving the patient. If the patient is wedged between the seat and the steering wheel, the seat may be slid back manually while rescuers support the patient. If the seat has become dislodged from the track, then the patient should be completely immobilized because this type of mechanical damage can result in severe physical injury. If the patient's legs are trapped, lifting the steering wheel away may also lift the dashboard and help to release the patient.

CUTTING A VEHICLE

If a patient must be **cut from a vehicle** (such as when the vehicle is on its side and access must be through a U-shaped flap in the roof), he or she should be warned of the noise and should be covered with a safety blanket (heavy aluminized). In some accidents, **air bags** may deploy with the movement of the patient or vehicle, resulting in danger to the patient and EMS personnel. If the air bags have not deployed, then the battery cables should be disconnected or cut (negative side first) to prevent deployment and personnel should avoid being in front of the path of deployment. EMS personnel should check for side air bags as well as front. The air bags should be deactivated before the steering column is moved (keeping in mind that deactivation can take up to 30 minutes), and care should be taken to avoid cutting or drilling into an air bag.

SEAT BELT PRETENSIONERS

Since the 1990s, vehicles have been equipped with **seat belt pretensioners** on three-point (shoulder harness) systems in the front and often also in the back. The purpose of seat belt pretensioners is to tighten any slack in the belts in an accident, pulling the person back into the seat and in the proper position for deployment of the air bag. Evidence of pretensioners is not always visible, although an accordion sleeve near the buckle end may be an indication. This sleeve compresses if the pretensioner fires. Although an undeployed pretensioner poses less threat to EMS personnel than an undeployed air bag, it can increase the risk of injury to the patient or EMS personnel, so the seat belt should be disconnected or cut immediately on access to the patient. If the patient was not wearing the seat belt on impact and the pretensioner fired, the seat belt will be tightly vertical along pillar B. If the seat belt pretensioner fired while being worn, it will be extended and will not be retractable.

TOOL KIT

Although large and heavy pieces of equipment, such as hydraulic rescue tools (including the Jaws of Life, cutters, spreaders, truck jacks, and rams), pneumatic tools, and come-along tools, are often used in vehicle extrication, a **tool kit** with simple hand tools should also be readily available. They may also be needed to access and safely remove a patient from a vehicle. Tools that may be needed for disassembly include adjustable wrenches, screwdrivers (flat and Phillips), flashlight, penlight, medical scissors, headlamp, pliers, bolt cutters, hammers, axes, crowbars, rescue knives (specially designed to cut through seat belts and clothing), and tin snips. Combination rescue tools are available that can be used for a variety of purposes, such as shutting off gas valves, prying open windows, and cutting through battery cables. Tool belt pouches are available to hold small tools that may be needed during an extrication.

CRIBBING AND CHOCKING

Cribbing and chocking are used to raise a vehicle and prevent it from rolling, such as when a patient is caught beneath a vehicle. **Cribbing** consists of 2×4 blocks and wedges and 4×4 blocks and wedges that are used to create crib boxes to hold an air bag. Cribs are usually made of Douglas fir or southern yellow pine, which can hold 500 psi and crush slowly. The cribbing is stacked with a 4-inch overhang (to allow for compression), and it should not exceed 48 inches in height. The crib box is put in place with the air bag on top. **Chocks** are large stepped wedges that are placed in front of or behind wheels to keep them from rolling when the air bag is inflated. As the air bag is slowly inflated, capture cribbing stacks are placed on both sides behind it to hold the vehicle when the air bag is deflated. Once the vehicle is elevated and secured, the air bag is deflated and the crib box is removed to allow room for the extrication of the patient.

VEHICLES POWERED BY ALTERNATIVE FUELS

Some vehicles are powered by **alternative fuels**, such as compressed natural gas (CNG) or liquefied natural gas (LNG), so EMS personnel should look for CNG/LNG logos, often on the right rear or near the refueling port or the right rear of the cab (semitruck). A "natural gas vehicle" warning may be located near the bottom of the rear doors. CNG tanks may be located behind the cabs in semi-trucks, and some may have additional saddle tanks. The power should be turned off, and the 12-volt battery positive and negative cables should be cut. The emergency shut-off valve should be located and turned off, although each tank can also be turned off manually. Electric vehicles pose the risk of stranded energy. Batteries should always be considered energized with a potential for high-voltage injury. Damaged lithium ion batteries that are leaking or sparking are at risk for thermal runaway (fire). The car battery should be shut down immediately. If the battery is damaged, the vehicle must be relocated at least 50 feet from any combustible material.

BUS EXTRICATION

Before accessing patients involved in a **bus crash,** the bus must be stabilized, especially if it is on its side or if it is upside down. If the engine is still running, a stop button is often located on the left side of the front panel. Access to the bus may be through the front door if possible. Access may also be through the front windshield (which can be removed through removal of the rubber locking strip that surrounds the window), side windows, the emergency exit door or window, the bathroom window, or an opening cut into the top of the vehicle. Removal of injured patients, usually on stretchers, from inside the vehicle often requires rapid triage and the assistance of multiple EMS personnel. If the vehicle remains upright but patients are completely or partially beneath the vehicle, they should be removed quickly because they may be crushed if the air suspension system deflates.

AIRCRAFT EXTRICATION

Communication is essential if EMS personnel are responding to an **aircraft crash site** because they need to know when the crash occurred, the type and size of the aircraft, the number of passengers and crew, reports of fire or explosion, and whether the aircraft is private, commercial, or military, as well as the status (fire, collapse) of any structure(s) that the aircraft may have impacted. For a small plane with the cabin still reasonably intact, extrication may be similar to a motor vehicle, but severe crashes in which the cabin is destroyed and large airplane crashes pose significantly different problems because passengers may have been thrown about inside or outside of the aircraft and seats and belongings and body parts may block access. Victims may lie in the roadway, so emergency vehicles must proceed with caution. Fire and explosions may be a severe risk, and rescuers may need to wait for fire suppression. Triage may begin outside of the aircraft while the aircraft (or the remains of the aircraft) is secured.

ADDITIONAL EXTRICATION CONSIDERATIONS
CONTROL ZONES

Part of the stabilization of the scene is ensuring that it is secure. An outer perimeter is established to block public and media access, and an inner perimeter is established immediately about the scene of the rescue and the working crew. Three **control zones** are established as follows:

- **Hot (coded red)**: This encompasses the inner perimeter and the crew as well as any area that is dangerous, such as an area contaminated by hazardous material or one in danger of a release of toxins.
- **Warm (coded orange)**: Area for trained personnel in support of those in the hot zone. Decontamination of patients, crew, and equipment is carried out in this zone.
- **Cold (coded yellow)**: This is the staging area and the command post (if necessary, for the emergent situation). No members of the public or media should be allowed in the cold zone.

Zones are usually established by placement of police cars and fire-line tape.

PATH OF LEAST RESISTANCE

The path of least resistance is an important concept to understand for rescues, especially if they involve fire and any products of combustion (smoke, heat, gas). Fire's path of least resistance is usually vertical and upward, although fire also spreads horizontally, especially if a vertical path is not available. It's for this reason that if there is a fire on the top floor of a building, the roof is breached to prevent horizontal spread. External factors, such as gusts of wind, can affect the path of least resistance. Water, on the other hand, also flows vertically, but downward and then horizontally if the downward flow is blocked. If the EMS provider is rescuing patients from a building, they will often be found near the path of least resistance, such as near a door or window. Patients should also be transported according to the path of least resistance, that is, the route that is the easiest and safest.

MULTISTEP RESCUE PROCESS

The multistep rescue process includes the following 10 steps:

1. **Preparation**: Training, readying equipment, and preparing for different types of rescues
2. **Response**: Using protocols for dispatch; contacting others, such as utility companies, which may have the necessary knowledge or equipment
3. **Situation size-up**: 360° site survey to identify hazards and determine the need for additional personnel or equipment (Determine if the situation is rescuer/equipment intensive.)
4. **Stabilization**: Establishing perimeters and control zones, monitoring hazardous atmosphere, carrying out lockout/tagout of industrial equipment
5. **Access**: Gaining access to the patient and providing emergent care
6. **Disentanglement**: Freeing the patient
7. **Removal**: Continuing critical and life support while assisting the patient to move or carrying the immobilized patient (Rapid extraction if his or her condition is life threatening.)
8. **Transport**: Transporting by various means with decontamination done as needed
9. **Scene security**: Police or others providing protection of the scene, crew, and patients
10. **Post-event analysis**: Reviewing the procedures performed and the problems encountered

CRITICAL INCIDENT STRESS MANAGEMENT (CISM)

Critical incident stress management (CISM) is a procedure to help people cope with stressful events, such as disasters, in order to reduce the incidence of **post-traumatic stress syndrome (PTSS)**.

-   **Defusing sessions** usually occur very early, sometimes during or immediately after a stressful event, and they are used to educate personnel who are actively involved about what to expect over the next few days and to provide guidance in handling their feelings and stress levels.
-   **Debriefing sessions** usually follow in one to three days and may be repeated periodically as needed. These sessions may include people who were directly involved as well as those who were indirectly involved. People are encouraged to express their emotions about the event. Critiquing the event or attempting to place blame is not productive as part of the CISM process.
-   **Follow-up** is done at the end of the process, usually after about a week, but this time frame can vary.

Mass Casualty and Terrorism

MULTIPLE-CASUALTY INCIDENTS VERSUS MASS-CASUALTY INCIDENTS

Multiple-casualty incidents involve more than one person, but different jurisdictions may quantify the total number of persons differently. It usually refers to the following:

- An incident involving at least three patients
- An incident involving only one jurisdiction and only one to three agencies (ambulance, fire department, and police)
- An incident requiring triage, but generally only primary triage
- Standards of care are maintained, and all patients not coded black (deceased) are transported for care

Mass-casualty incidents also involve more than one person, but may involve much larger numbers—dozens, hundreds, or thousands.

- Often involves multiple jurisdictions and agencies
- Requires triage but may also involve separate waiting areas for color-coded individuals and secondary triage
- Standards of care may be modified, and patients coded black (expectant) and not expected to live may be left in the field and/or receive delayed care if they are still living after the red- and yellow-coded individuals are transported

ROLE OF THE TRANSPORTATION OFFICER IN A MASS-CASUALTY INCIDENT

During a mass-casualty event, the **transportation officer** must maintain constant communication with hospitals and trauma centers, triage officers, police, ground ambulance services, and air medical transport services. The transportation officer controls the flow of patients for treatment and must determine where to route patients in order to prevent a backlog at the receiving facility. They must also coordinate incoming and outgoing ambulances in the transportation staging area. The transportation officer must obtain information about each facility's surge capacity and the number and types of patients the facility is prepared to care for. The transportation officer must also coordinate air medical transport flights and determine, with the triage officer, which patients to transport by air according to their severity of injuries, availability of treatment options, and appropriate levels of care. Speed of transportation and care is often critical in a mass-casualty incident because delays often result in increased death rates.

ROLE OF TRIAGE

In a mass-casualty incident related to terrorism or a disaster, **rapid triage** and tagging must occur and patients must be sorted according to priority for transportation or field treatment. Because of the large numbers of casualties, triage should begin with the first patient encountered, proceeding from one to another. According to some plans, patients who are alive but expected to die are coded red, but this can result in overtriage, with too many red-coded individuals having to be transported and/or treated, resulting in patients dying during the wait. With other plans, patients expected to die are black-coded as "expectant" and left in the field or left aside until red- and yellow-coded individuals are transported and/or treated. If patients are undertriaged (such as patients who should be coded red being coded yellow instead) this can also result in increased deaths while other patients are waiting for transport or treatment.

GUIDANCE FOR INCREASING SURVIVAL RATES IN MASS-CASUALTY EVENTS

Terrorist or other attacks that involve active shooters or improvised explosive devices (IEDs) often result in injuries similar to those encountered in combat situations in which the most common causes of death are extremity hemorrhage, tension pneumothorax, and airway obstruction. The **THREAT acronym** provides guidance for dealing with these situations in the following ways:

- **Threat suppression**: Use of police protection, ballistic vests, concealment, cover, and situational awareness. One concern is that most of the protective gear available to emergency medical personnel is for ballistics rather than explosive devices.
- **Hemorrhage control**: Use of tourniquets (military style) and hemostatic dressings (QuikClot) to control bleeding.
- **Rapid Extrication to safety**: Move patients and personnel out of the danger zone to prevent further injuries.
- **Assessment by medical providers**: Includes provision of a nasopharyngeal airway or upright seating and leaning forward for airway compromise and spinal precautions.
- **Transport to definitive care**: Medical treatment should continue during transport.

SAFETY CONSIDERATIONS ASSOCIATED WITH ACTIVE SHOOTERS AND TERRORIST BOMB ATTACKS

With **active shooters**, standard protocol has been for emergency response services to wait until the police have removed the threat and secured the area before moving in to care for victims; however, this delay in treatment may result in death, so some authorities are now recommending that emergency response personnel enter the scene with police while wearing appropriate protective equipment, although this does pose some risk, especially with additional shooters or a secondary attack.

With a **terrorist bombing** and improvised explosive devices (IEDs), situational awareness is critical because multiple explosive devices (some undetonated) may be at the scene. IEDs may be inside backpacks, suitcases, and packages left unattended, and in emergency situations innocent people often drop backpacks and packages and run away, making it difficult to tell identify a threat. Additionally, attackers wearing suicide vests or belts may mix in with other victims or people escaping the blast area.

BOMB THREAT STANDOFF RECOMMENDATIONS

Threat	Explosive capacity (lb)	Mandatory evacuation distance (ft)	Preferred evacuation distance (ft)	Shelter-in-place zone (ft)
Pipe bomb	5	70	1200+	71–1199
Suicide bomber	20	110	1700+	111–1699
Suitcase/Briefcase	50	150	1850+	151–1849
Automobile	500	320	1900+	321–1899
SUV/Van	1000	400	2400+	401–2399
Small truck	4000	640	3800+	641–3799
Container truck	10,000	860	5100+	861–5099
Semitrailer	60,000	1570	9300+	1571–9299

Source: U.S. Department of Homeland Security.

B-NICE HAZARDOUS MATERIAL (HAZMAT) INCIDENTS ASSOCIATED WITH TERRORIST ATTACKS

Category	Response
B—Biological (bacteria, viruses, fungi, toxins)	Inhalation type—evacuate for 80 feet, shut down air-handling systems, wear appropriate PPE and SCBA, and avoid contamination. Visible agent—decontaminate with soap and water. Symptoms may vary but are usually delayed.
N—Nuclear/ Radiological	Inhalation type (most common)—Isolate/Secure the area, avoid smoke/fumes, stay upwind, and use PPE and SCBA. Isolate victims and decontaminate as appropriate. Symptoms are usually delayed.
I—Incendiary	Be on alert for multiple devices and sabotaged fire suppression equipment. Symptoms include burns, pain, and trauma.
C—Chemical	Isolate/Secure the area, decontaminate victims with soap and water, and be on alert for chemical dispersal devices. Approach toward uphill and upwind. Isolate symptomatic patients from others. Symptoms vary but may include burns, blistering, vomiting, breathing difficulty, and neurological damage.
E—Explosives	Be alert for secondary devices, undetonated devices, and secondary hazards (unstable buildings and debris). Remove victims from the area, secure the perimeter, and stage away from the incident area. Decontaminate as necessary. Symptoms include burns, amputations, cuts, and penetrating and blunt trauma.

"ALL-HAZARDS" SAFETY APPROACH TO MASS-CASUALTY INCIDENTS

The "all-hazards" safety approach to mass-casualty incidents aims to provide plans that can be used to deal with all types of hazards (natural disasters, terrorist attacks, and mass-casualty incidents) as well as encompassing the four components of emergency management: mitigation, preparedness, response, and recovery. Organizations in an area coordinate to develop joint action plans that can be activated in response to incidents, with the chain of command clearly outlined. This approach lowers costs to individual organizations and provides for a faster and more effective response. However, although the basic structure may be the same for responding to all hazards, there are inevitable differences between (for example) a terrorist attack with active shooters and a natural disaster, such as a hurricane, which can be anticipated and mitigated to some degree. For this reason, modifying existing incident action plans to meet the needs of a situation is essential.

TREATING TERRORISTS AND CRIMINALS

In mass-casualty incidents, **terrorists and criminals** involved in the incident may be injured and require treatment, and EMS personnel may feel conflicted about providing treatment when others have been injured or killed, but it's important to provide treatment to terrorists and criminals the same as any other individuals both because they are in need of help and because their survival may be critical to identifying co-conspirators and to providing reasons for the attack.

However, these individuals may pose risks to emergency medical personnel, so they should be examined while under police guard. The individual's hands should be examined first to check for weapons and detonators and secured (with handcuffs, if possible). Clothes should be examined and removed very carefully in case the person is wearing a suicide device of some type. Emergency medical personnel should also be aware that the individual may be feigning injury or unconsciousness.

EMS Regulations

EMS HISTORY

Historically, the **first use of an ambulance** was in the Siege of Málaga in Spain in 1487, when horse-drawn wagons were used to carry the wounded to safety. Military ambulances became more common in Europe throughout the following centuries. Napoleon Bonaparte assigned battlefield vehicles and attendants in 1793. The first ambulance service in the United States was instituted by the US army in 1865 in Cincinnati, followed by an ambulance service in New York just four years later. Hospital-based ambulance services increased in the 1900s, but many hospital ambulance services shut down during World War II, so fire and police departments filled the roles. At this time, there were no laws regarding minimum training for ambulance personnel. Following World War II, the use of ambulance services increased, but the quality was often poor until basic training standards were developed in 1968 along with the 911 emergency system. The **first paramedic program** was developed in 1969. The EMS Systems Act was passed in 1973, the EMS for Children Act in 1983, and the Trauma Care Systems Planning and Development Act in 1990. In 1991, standards and benchmarks for ambulance services were established by the Commission on Accreditation of Ambulance Services.

EMS SYSTEMS

The **National Highway Traffic Safety Administration** (**NHTSA**) is the lead agency for coordinating and promoting evidence-based emergency medical services (EMS) (fire based, third service, and hospital based) and the 911 system. The **public safety answering point** (**PSAP**) is the designated call-receiving site that directs calls to the appropriate emergency services. Each state defines the scope of practice, licensure, and credentialing for prehospital personnel and sets education standards based on national EMS standards. The EMS provider of any level is expected to maintain certification through maintenance of skills and continuing education and should exhibit professional behavior, including working with integrity and empathy, being an effective member of a team, showing respect and tact, maintaining a professional appearance, communicating effectively, and advocating for patients. The provider must be alert to patient safety and recognize that most errors result from skills-based, rules-based, and knowledge-based failures. Error reduction requires the use of decision aids and protocols, asking for assistance when appropriate, questioning assumptions, and making debriefing calls.

ROLES AND RESPONSIBILITIES OF EMS PERSONNEL

Roles and responsibilities of EMS personnel include the following:

- Maintain the readiness of all equipment, including disinfecting, packaging, and storing.
- Monitor personal safety, patient safety, and the safety of others on the scene.
- Evaluate the scene for additional resources when indicated.
- Gain access to the patient only when it is safe to do so.
- Perform an assessment of the patient's condition and needs.
- Provide emergency medical care as needed (or until additional resources arrive).
- Provide emotional support to the patient, family, and other providers.
- Maintain the continuity of care.
- Ensure that medical and legal standards are upheld and that patient privacy is protected.
- Communicate with others and maintain community relations.
- Practice professional behavior (integrity, self-motivation, self-confidence, tact, respect, and professional appearance).
- Maintain certification and meet continuing education requirements.

NATIONAL EMS EDUCATION AGENDA FOR THE FUTURE: A SYSTEMS APPROACH

The National EMS Education Agenda for the Future: A Systems Approach proposed an education system for EMS with five primary components, establishing the following goals for 2020:

- **Core content**: Core content to be developed by the EMS medical community, educators, and providers under leadership of the National Highway Traffic Safety Administration (NHTSA) to ensure consistency of content and reciprocity of certification. The core content should be tied to licensure and accreditation.
- **Scope-of-practice model**: National models to be used by states for all levels of EMS certification/licensure.
- **Education standards**: Standards that are developed by EMS educators with input from the medical community and regulators and that are peer reviewed.
- **Education program accreditation**: A single national accreditation agency will develop standards and guidelines.
- **EMS certification:** Four levels of national certification with different educational requirements, standards, scopes of practice, and certification:
  - (1) Entry-level emergency medical responder (EMR)
  - (2) Emergency medical technician (EMT)
  - (3) Advanced EMT (AEMT)
  - (4) Paramedic

Patient Safety and Quality Improvement

PATIENT SAFETY AND HIGH-RISK SITUATIONS

Up to 250,000 patients die each year because of medical errors. Patients are especially at risk of further injury or death in **high-risk situations** and activities such as the following:

- **Hand-off**: A standard procedure, such as **SBAR**, should be used.
    S = Situation: Overview of current situation and important issues
    B = Background: Important history and issues leading to current situation
    A = Assessment: Summary of important facts and condition
    R = Recommendation: Actions needed
- **Communications**: Problems may result in delayed or inadequate care, wrong address, or wrong destination.
- **Dropping**: Patients can be easily dropped if the gurney isn't positioned properly or if too few personnel are involved in transport.
- **Ambulance crashes**: Unnecessary speeding and failing to stop at intersections are the most common causes of ambulance crashes.
- **Inadequate spinal immobilization**: If unsure, it's always best to immobilize.
- **Medication errors**: Administration of wrong medication, wrong mode of administration, and wrong dosage.

QUALITY IMPROVEMENT

Quality improvement requires that an organization or system continually evaluates processes and outcomes and takes measures to improve the quality of care. The focus of quality improvement is on patient safety in access, provision of care, transport, and hand-off. Errors are often related to these different types of failures:

- **Skills-based**: Includes slips and mistakes. Slips occur when the EMS provider has the correct intent but does not carry out an action as intended, such as mistakenly using the wrong piece of equipment. Mistakes occur when the EMS provider has an incorrect intention that leads to incorrect action.
- **Rules-based**: The EMS provider incorrectly applies a rule, applies a bad or wrong rule, or fails to apply the correct rules. For example, an EMS provider is injured because of failing to assess safety before approaching a patient.
- **Knowledge-based**: The EMS provider's knowledge is not adequate for the situation.

EMS personnel can help reduce errors by debriefing, constantly reevaluating and questioning assumptions, using established protocols and decision aids, and asking for assistance when needed.

CONTINUOUS QUALITY IMPROVEMENT (CQI)

Continuous quality improvement (CQI) emphasizes the organization and systems and processes within that organization rather than emphasizing individuals. It recognizes internal customers (staff) and external customers (patients) and uses data to improve processes. CQI represents the concept that most processes can be improved. CQI uses the scientific method of experimentation to meet needs and improve services and uses various tools, such as brainstorming, multivoting, storyboarding, and meetings. **Core concepts** include the following:

- Quality and success are meeting or exceeding internal and external customers' needs and expectations.
- Problems relate to processes, and variations in processes lead to variations in results.
- Change can be made in small steps.

Steps to CQI include the following:

1. Forming a knowledgeable team
2. Identifying and defining measures used to determine success
3. Brainstorming strategies for change
4. Planning, collecting, and using data as part of making decisions
5. Testing changes and revising or refining as needed

Research and Evidence-Based Practice

DATA COLLECTION AND RESEARCH

Research is especially important in identifying the need for changes in procedures and protocols in order to improve patient outcomes. Research depends on the gathering of data. **Data collection** may include direct observations, surveys, interviews, and various other sources of information, such as documents and audiovisual materials. **Literature research** requires a comprehensive evaluation of current (≤5 years) and/or historical information. Most literature research begins with an internet search of databases, which provides listings of books, journals, and other materials on specific topics. Databases vary in content, and many contain only a reference listing with or without an abstract, so once the listing is obtained, the researcher must do a further search (publisher, library, etc.) to locate the material. Some databases require a subscription, but access is often available through educational or healthcare institutions. In order to search effectively, the researcher should begin by writing a brief explanation of the research to help identify possible keywords and synonyms to use as search words.

METHODS OF DATA COLLECTION

When developing **data collection procedures** to determine needs, the following must be considered: the purpose of the data collection, the audience for which the data are intended, the types of questions to be answered, the scope of the research, and the resources available to carry out data collection. Methods of collection and subsequent issues regarding those procedures are discussed below:

- **Direct observation**: Observers must be selected and trained on how to observe and when and how to record observations.
- **Interviews**: Interview questions must be developed and validated, and the interviewers must be given practice time.
- **Questionnaires**: The type of questionnaire, the questions, and the Likert scale must be determined as well as the method of distribution (one-on-one, group, email, internet).
- **Record review**: A form or checklist should be developed to guide record review, and the records should be selected based on criteria established for the research.
- **Secondary analysis**: The databases to be mined should be selected, and the criteria for the research should be established, including keywords, time frames, and populations.

EVIDENCE-BASED DECISION-MAKING

Although traditional medical practice has been based on knowledge, intuition, and judgment, these practices have not always been supported by evidence. **Evidence-based decision-making** results in best practices based on best evidence. Steps include the following:

1. Formulating a question regarding treatment and/or procedures
2. Conducting a search of the appropriate medical literature, often beginning with the search of an online database to find research that is related to the question
3. Determining the validity (measure of accuracy) and reliability (consistency) of the evidence
4. Evaluating the level of evidence (1-5, 1 being the most reliable)
5. Assessing data (information) to determine if they apply to current needs
6. Drawing up a plan for change with input from all staff members
7. Implementing changes
8. Monitoring changes and outcomes

Workplace Safety and Wellness

STRESS MANAGEMENT

The EMS provider must often deal with **stressful incidents**, such as dangerous situations (storm conditions, gunshots, falling debris); critically ill patients; unpleasant sights, sounds, and odors; multi-patient incidents; and angry/upset patients, family members, and bystanders. The EMS provider should not argue or become defensive but should remain calm and supportive, allowing the patient to express his or her feelings and trying to defuse the situation while administering medical care and cooperating with other first responders. If a patient has no pulse or respirations and does not have a valid do-not-resuscitate (DNR) order, the EMS provider should attempt resuscitation unless doing so puts the provider at risk; the injuries are not compatible with life; or obvious signs of death are present, such as tissue decay, livor mortis, which is discoloration in the lowermost blood vessels from pooled blood shortly after death, or rigor mortis, which is stiffening of the joints that occurs within 2-6 hours of death (verified by checking two or more joints). After 24-48 hours of rigor mortis, the muscles become flaccid.

WARNING SIGNS OF STRESS

Warning signs of stress often begin with difficulty sleeping and nightmares about work, loss of appetite, and lack of interest in usual activities, including work and intimacy. The individual may feel increasingly sad and depressed and may have difficulty concentrating, making decisions, and carrying out tasks. The individual may also begin to isolate from others and exhibit irritability with coworkers, family, and friends. Some individuals develop physical symptoms related to stress, such as stomach upset, headaches, nausea, and high blood pressure (BP), whereas others may experience panic attacks. Some individuals may try to self-medicate with alcohol or drugs. When experiencing the warning signs of stress, the individual should talk about the problems with someone trusted, such as a physician, coworker, supervisor, or family member, and he or she may need to seek assistance from a professional counselor. Lifestyle changes, such as decreasing the use of alcohol or drugs, exercising regularly, and practicing relaxation exercises, may help to relieve stress.

STRESS REACTIONS

Stress reactions include the following:

- **Acute stress reaction**: This reaction usually occurs quickly (minutes to hours) in response to an event that is stressful (such as the death of a child or a multiple-casualty incident). The individual may experience physical symptoms (with the release of adrenaline) such as rapid pulse, nausea, chest tightness, headache, fast respirations, and increased perspiration. An acute stress reaction usually recedes quickly, but it may persist for weeks in some individuals.
- **Delayed stress reaction**: Although the individual may cope well with a stressful event initially, months later, the person may begin to have nightmares, anxiety, and other indications of post-traumatic stress.
- **Cumulative stress reaction**: This type of stress reaction occurs when the individual has repeated stressors (either in the workplace or in his or her personal life) that cause repeated acute stress reactions, resulting in various physical and psychological problems. This is especially common in EMS personnel.

PREVENTION OF RESPONSE-RELATED INJURIES

Prevention of response-related injuries includes the following:

- **Infectious diseases**: Use PPE and understand the spread of infectious diseases—air (coughing), direct contact (blood, vomitus, other body fluids), needlestick, contaminated food/equipment, and sexual transmission. Maintain current immunizations.
- **Personal habits**: Obtain adequate sleep, nutrition, and exercise. Avoid excessive alcohol and tobacco.
- **Environmental hazards**: Conduct a 360° assessment. Note traffic hazards, the vehicle's condition, fire, leaking fluids, downed power lines, hazardous materials (look for placards and warning symbols; avoid the area until it is cleared). Use PPE and respirators as indicated.
- **Violence**: Defuse situations, make a safe response (with the assistance of law enforcement), and use restraints if necessary, for dangerous or violent individuals.
- **Collisions**: Drive safely; avoid speeding and driving through stop signs and red lights when possible. Wear seat belts and/or safety harnesses.

PRINCIPLES OF BODY MECHANICS

Basic principles of body mechanics include the following:

- Avoid reaching overhead or for prolonged periods of time or more than 20 inches away.
- Avoid pulling—push, roll, or slide instead.
- Avoid lifting—push, roll, or slide instead.
- Lift with leg muscles, not with the back.
- Hold weight close to the body rather than at arm's length.
- Flex at the hips and knees, not the waist.
- Carry patients head first upstairs and feet first downstairs.
- Maintain a straight back and avoid twisting.
- Assess weight and recognize limitations in lifting/carrying.
- Get help when necessary, and communicate every step with your partner ("Lift on the count of three").
- Maintain a firm base of support with feet apart (shoulder width) to stabilize your stance.
- Maintain the line of gravity (the imaginary line between your center of gravity and the ground) within the base of support.
- Position yourself close to an object that is to be lifted or carried.
- Lift patients from stable ground.

MOVING AND LIFTING PATIENTS

Techniques for moving patients include the following:

- **Direct ground lift**: Use only for lightweight individuals with no suspected spinal injuries. Three EMS providers line up on one side of the patient, and each kneels on the same knee. The EMS provider at the head places one arm under the patient's neck and shoulder and the other arm under the patient's lower back. The middle provider places his or her arms above and below the patient's waist, and the provider at the patient's feet places his or her arms under the knees and lower legs. On the count of three, they roll the patient onto their knees and toward their chests. On the count of three, they stand and move the patient.
- **Power lift**: Place feet shoulder width apart and pointing slightly outward; tighten the back and abdominal muscles. Squat down as though sitting. Place hands 10 inches apart with the palms upward (power grip) while grasping the stretcher and lift with the upper body becoming vertical before the hips rise.
- **Extremity lift**: Requires two EMS providers. One provider squats at the patient's head and another is at one side by the patient's knees. The provider at the head folds the patient's arms across the chest and grasps the patient by wrapping both arms around the torso under the patient's arms and grasping the patient's wrists. The second provider slides his or her hands beneath the patient's knees and lower legs, and together they stand and lift the patient.
- **Squat lift**: Requires two EMS providers. One provider squats with the back straight and the weak foot slightly forward at the head of patient, and the other provider is in the same position at the patient's feet. Grasp the patient's upper body as for the extremity lift and grasp the patient's feet. Both EMS providers push up with the stronger foot and lift with the upper body becoming vertical before the hips rise.
- **Logroll**: Used to position carrying devices under the patient and for some transfers; it requires two EMS providers positioned on the same side of the patient. Place the patient's arm on the side that he or she is being turned to above his or her head or over the chest. Place the patient's other arm across his or her chest. If on the ground, squat close to the patient. The provider at the patient's head reaches across the patient and grasps his or her shoulders and trunk while the second provider grasps his or her trunk and legs. On the count of three, they turn the patient in one smooth move.
- **Draw-sheet transfer**: Requires four EMS providers with two positioned on one side of the patient and two positioned on the other side but on the opposite side of the bed or stretcher to which the patient will be transferred. The logroll technique is used to place a draw sheet under the patient. Providers on both sides roll the edges of the draw sheet until the edges are close to the patient. On the count of three, they lift the patient slightly and move the patient across to the bed.

Occupational Safety

OCCUPATIONAL SAFETY AND HEALTH ADMINISTRATION (OSHA)

The Occupational Safety and Health Administration (OSHA) is part of the U.S. Department of Labor, and it is charged with ensuring safe, healthful working conditions and setting and enforcing workplace standards. OSHA covers most employers in the private sector, but state and federal safety regulations also generally conform to OSHA standards. Employers must provide safety training, inform workers of chemical hazards, and provide required PPE. OSHA must be notified of a workplace-related death within 8 hours and a workplace-related injury that results in hospitalization, the loss of an eye, or amputation within 24 hours. Workers may file a complaint about workplace conditions with OSHA and request an inspection. OSHA's Whistleblower Protection Program prohibits retaliation by the employer. OSHA provides Hazardous Waste Operations and Emergency Response Standard (HAZWOPER) training courses (8-hour, 24-hour, 40-hour, and refresher) for first responders. OSHA has established regulations and guidelines that are industry specific. For example, OSHA has regulations regarding EMS. OSHA requires that hazardous material be color coded, with red indicating danger; yellow, caution; orange, warning; and fluorescent orange/orange-red, biological hazard.

> **Review Video: Intro to OSHA**
> Visit mometrix.com/academy and enter code: 913559

SAFETY DATA SHEETS (SDSs)

Safety data sheets (SDSs), formerly known as material safety data sheets (MSDSs), explain how to handle caustic substances in the event of an accident or injury and provide pertinent information on the composition and toxic effects of chemicals in a lab. SDSs outline the proper storage of chemicals, procedures for the cleanup and dumping of caustic substances, procedures in the event of a chemical spill or injury, and the proper locations in the facility for cleanup. SDSs should also contain information indicating which substances may cause allergic effects or asthma from contact or inhalation. Emergency rescue services should obtain SDSs for common chemicals and products. Manufacturers and suppliers should have SDSs on file and can be contacted for copies. The OSHA/ Environmental Protection Agency (EPA) Occupational Chemical Database provides links for SDSs for some products. SDSs are available from various other sources, including the Toxicology Data Network (TOXNET) and poison control centers. There are also pathogen safety data sheets for biological hazards.

HAZARDOUS MATERIALS, EXPOSURE, AND ABSORPTION

Hazardous materials are any materials that may cause harm to humans or animals by themselves or through interaction with something else. **Hazardous materials** may be any of the following:

- **Chemical**: Blister agents, blood agents, choking agents, nerve agents, asphyxiants, or irritants that can enter the body through inhalation, absorption, ingestion, or injection
- **Radiological**: Nuclear material and radioactive substances (alpha/beta particles)
- **Physical/Biological**: Infectious wastes, blood and other body fluids, and biotoxins

Almost any material or substance can be classified as hazardous depending on various factors such as its location, amount, and interactions. **Exposure** occurs when a person/animal comes in contact with the hazardous material, and contamination is the residue resulting from exposure. **Absorption** is the method by which hazardous material enters the bloodstream. Exposure and contamination may result in an immediate response (blistering, itching, and pain) or a delayed response (nausea, vomiting, cancer, and lung disease).

CLASSIFICATION OF HAZARDOUS WASTE

The Environmental Protection Agency (EPA) **classifies hazardous wastes** according to the following characteristics:

- **Ignitable**: Liquids and nonliquids that can ignite and cause fires with flash points of <60 °C (140 °F)
- **Corrosive**: Based on pH (<2 or >12.5) or its ability to corrode steel
- **Reactive**: Wastes that are unstable, may react with water, may result in toxic gases, or may explode
- **Toxic**: Heavy metal compounds that are harmful if ingested or absorbed

Wastes may also be classified as **listed wastes**. These include wastes from manufacturing and industrial processes. Hazardous wastes are often produced in manufacturing, nuclear power plants (nuclear wastes), and healthcare facilities (needles and materials contaminated with body fluids). Nuclear wastes are classified as mixed waste because they contain a radioactive component as well as a hazardous component. Hazardous wastes can result in disease (such as from needle punctures), injury (from fire and explosions), and death (from toxic exposure and disease).

HAZARDOUS WASTE SITE CHARACTERIZATION

The purpose of hazardous waste site characterization is to identify hazards and select the appropriate PPE. The team leader is responsible for the assessment, but he or she may request assistance from outside experts, such as chemists. The three **steps to hazardous waste site characterization** include the following:

1. **Off-site characterization**: Gather information/data before personnel enter the site, including the location, a description of the activities, the duration of the event, terrain information (photographs, maps), habitation/population data, accessibility, paths of least resistance, and properties of any hazardous materials/substances. Conduct the needed interviews and review of records. Perimeter reconnaissance is done with observations, air sampling, and development of a preliminary site map.
2. **On-site survey**: Verify the information gathered from perimeter reconnaissance, survey the area and situation, note potential exposure to hazardous materials (dust, liquid, dead animals, gas) and safety hazards (obstacles, terrain, poisonous plants), and develop a site safety plan. The entry team should have at least four members: two to enter and two for outside support who can enter the site in an emergency.
3. **Ongoing monitoring**: Monitoring should be continuous.

CHEMICAL HAZARDOUS WASTE MATERIALS

Types of chemical hazardous waste materials include the following:

- **Blister agents**: Include sulfur mustard (mustard gas) and nitrogen mustard, which are both highly toxic. Exposure by inhalation, contact, or ingestion results in skin (erythema and blistering) and eye irritation and injury to the respiratory system as well as bone marrow suppression and gastrointestinal and neurological damage. The patient should be decontaminated within 1 to 2 minutes by flushing the eyes with water for up to 20 minutes and removing clothing and showering with soap (if available) and water for 20 minutes. Rescuers should use a self-contained breathing apparatus (SCBA), PPE (including eye protection), and chemical-protective gloves.
- **Asphyxiants**: Gas exposure (such as by butane, helium, and propane) lowers oxygen levels and results in suffocation. Patients require oxygen administration and may need CPR. This is especially a risk in confined spaces. Rescuers should use an SCBA.
- **Blood agents**: These include cyanide chloride, hydrogen cyanide, and arsine. Exposure by inhalation or ingestion. They prevent oxygen transfer from blood to cells. The patient may need oxygen and the antidote. Rescuers should use an SCBA.
- **Carcinogens**: Agents such as asbestos, nickel compounds, and ionizing radiation that result in genetic mutation and cancer. There are various types of exposure. Patients must be removed from exposure. The rescuer must wear adequate PPE, and in some cases, he or she should use a mask or SCBA.
- **Choking agents**: Often, a chemical weapon is used (ammonia, chlorine) that is designed to inhibit breathing and incapacitate the person. Exposure is by inhalation, contact, or ingestion (rare). They may be corrosive to the skin and result in fluid in the lungs, leading to suffocation. Patients require supportive treatment and oxygen. Rescuers should use PPE and SCBA for most agents.
- **Convulsants/Nerve agents**: These include hydrazine and strychnine. Exposure may be by inhalation, contact, and ingestion. The severity of convulsions and nervous system impairment is dose related. Patients require supportive treatment. Rescuers need SCBA and protective suits (according to the exposure level of the agent).

HAZARD SIGNS AND SYMBOLS

Sign/Symbol	Interpretation
	Flame: Includes flammable, self-heating, or self-reactive materials and gases.
	Corrosion: Includes substances that can cause skin burns, metal corrosion, and eye damage.
	Health hazard: Includes carcinogens, toxic substances, and respiratory irritants.
	Poison: Includes materials, gases, or substances that are extremely toxic and may result in death or severe illness.
	Irritant: Includes materials, gases, or substances that are irritants to the skin, eyes, and/or respiratory tract, are acutely toxic, or have a narcotic effect.
	Biohazard: Includes biological substances, such as body fluids, that pose a threat to humans. Appears on sharps containers that hold contaminated needles.

Infection Control

DISEASE PREVENTION

CDC ISOLATION GUIDELINES

The **2007 CDC Guideline for Isolation Precautions** includes the standard precautions that apply to all patients and transmission-based precautions for those with known or suspected infections.

Standard precautions should be used for all patients because all body fluids (sweat, urine, feces, blood, and sputum) and non-intact skin and mucous membranes may be infected. Standard precautions include the following:

- **Hand hygiene**: Use an alcohol-based hand rub or wash with soap and water before and after each patient contact and after any contact with body fluids and contaminated items. Always use soap and water when hands are visibly soiled.
- **Protective equipment**: Use personal protective equipment (PPE), such as gloves, gowns, and masks, eye protection, and/or face shields, when anticipating contact with body fluids or contaminated skin.
- **Respiratory hygiene/Cough etiquette**: Use source-control measures, such as covering cough, disposing of tissues, using a surgical mask on the person coughing or on staff to prevent inhalation of droplets, and properly disposing of dressings and used equipment. Wash hands after contacting respiratory secretions. Maintain a distance of >3 feet from a coughing person when possible.
- **Sharps**: Dispose of sharps, such as needles, carefully in sharps containers. Do not recap needles.

Transmission-based precautions should be used for those with known or suspected infections as well as those with excessive wound drainage, other discharge, or fecal incontinence. Transmission-based precautions include the following:

- **Contact**: Use PPE, including gown and gloves, for all contacts with the patient or the patient's immediate environment.
- **Droplet**: Appropriate for influenza, streptococcus infection, pertussis, rhinovirus, and adenovirus and pathogens that remain viable and infectious for only short distances. Use a mask while caring for the patient. Maintain the patient at a distance of >3 feet away from other patients (with a curtain separating them in an emergency department). Use a patient mask if transporting a patient.
- **Airborne**: Appropriate for measles, chickenpox, tuberculosis, severe acute respiratory syndrome [SARS] and COVID-19 because pathogens remain viable and infectious for long distances. Use ≥N95 respirators (or masks) while caring for the patient. The patient should be placed in an airborne infection isolation room (with negative air pressure if possible) in an emergency department.

PERSONAL PROTECTIVE EQUIPMENT (PPE)

Personal protective equipment (PPE) should be readily available in the appropriate sizes for each EMS individual.

- **Gowns**: Should be worn for risk of splash or spray with body fluids (severe bleeding, childbirth) and should be fluid resistant.
- **Eye protectors**: Should be worn for risk of splash or spray with body fluids or contact with debris, such as at a worksite or in a collapsing building. Goggles should fit snugly and have antifog features. (Prescription eyeglasses do not take the place of goggles.)
- **Face shields**: Provide protection for face, eyes, nose, and mouth. These are preferred to goggles when there is risk of spray or splash of body fluids. They should wrap around and cover the forehead and extend to below the chin.
- **Masks**: Protect the nose and mouth from fluids and particles and should be fluid resistant, fit snugly, and have a flexible nosepiece.
- **Respirators** (such as N95, N99, and N100): Protect the nose, mouth, and airway passages exposed to hazardous or infectious aerosols, including bacteria and viruses (tuberculosis [TB], measles, COVID-19).

HAND HYGIENE AND GLOVES

Hand hygiene should be done before eating, before and after direct contact with a patient's skin, after contact with any body fluids, after contact with inanimate objects in the patient's immediate vicinity, when moving hands from a dirty to a clean area, after removing gloves, and after using the restroom.

Hand hygiene is carried out in the following two manners:

- **Antiseptic soaps/detergents**: For visible soiling, after exposure to diarrhea stool or a patient with diarrhea, before eating, and after using the restroom. Wet hands, apply product, rub hands together vigorously for 15 seconds, covering all surfaces, rinse hands with water, and use a disposable towel to dry them.
- **Alcohol-based hand sanitizers** (the most effective way to kill bacteria): For all other situations. Apply product and rub hands together, including between the fingers, for about 20 seconds until the skin surfaces are dry.

Gloves must be worn when touching any body fluids, nonintact skin, open wounds, or mucous membranes (eyes, mouth, nose); gloves should be changed when moving from a dirty area to a clean one or from one patient to another.

IMMUNIZATIONS FOR EMS PERSONNEL

The Centers for Disease Control and Prevention (CDC) recommends the following **immunizations** for all healthcare workers, including EMS personnel:

- **Hepatitis B**: Three-dose series (now, in one month, and five months later) followed by an anti-HBs serologic test 30-60 days after the third immunization
- **Measles, mumps, rubella (MMR)**: Two-dose series with the second immunization at least 28 days after the first for those born during or after 1957 and those born before 1957 without proof of immunity
- **Varicella (chickenpox)**: Two doses, four weeks apart (A combined MMRV immunization is available.)
- **Influenza**: Annually
- **Tetanus, diphtheria, and pertussis (Tdap)**: One time, with a tetanus (TD) booster every 10 years (The TD injection does not protect against pertussis (whooping cough).)
- **Meningococcal**: One dose

Screening for **tuberculosis** with a chest x-ray or skin test is also recommended.

Documentation

MINIMUM DATA SETS

Minimum data sets are the minimum data specifically required for EMS services. These consist of the following:

- **Patient information**: This derives from the assessment including the patient's primary complaint and the findings during the initial assessment—the patient's name and address; vital signs (blood pressure [BP], pulse [P], and respiration rate [R]); and descriptions of any wounds, injuries, pain, or other symptoms. The patient's demographics (age, gender, ethnic background) should be noted as well as any other identifying or essential information.
- **Administrative information**: This includes the time of the initial report, time the EMS unit was notified, time of arrival at the incident, time of leaving the scene, time of arrival at the destination (hospital, trauma center), and time of hand-off.
- **Accurate/Synchronous clocks**: All members of the EMS system should use accurate and synchronous clocks so that they all are set to the same time to ensure there is no disparity in time reporting.

PREHOSPITAL CARE REPORT

The prehospital care report serves as a legal document to show that emergent care was provided. It describes the condition of the patient upon EMS arrival at the scene, interventions provided, and changes in the patient's condition; it is essential to ensure continuity of care. The documenting EMS provider may be called in to legal proceedings. The **prehospital care report** may also be used for educational purposes, such as through debriefing and case review. Additionally, the report is used administratively as the basis for billing as well as for the collection of data for research and evaluation of continuous quality improvement. Required elements of documentation include the time of events (receipt of call, arrival at incident, time of transport, arrival at destination), assessment findings (vital signs, injuries, bleeding, mental status), emergent care, changes in the patient's condition, response to the treatment provided, scene observations (specific place/area), hazards, and disposition of patient (care refusal, transportation, hand-off). Documentation may be on paper or may be done electronically and may combine checkboxes and narrative reports. **Run data** (or ambulance run report data) are those data elements that are required for reporting each run.

NARRATIVE DOCUMENTATION IN THE PREHOSPITAL CARE REPORT

With **narrative documentation**, the EMS provider should take care not to repeat the same information already provided in checkboxes. The provider should describe what was observed directly rather than the conclusions based on those observations and should record all pertinent information and observations, avoiding non-standardized abbreviations and radio codes, which may be misunderstood or misinterpreted. Any pertinent negatives, such as patient or family complaints, must be documented. If the incident has legal implications, such as in the case of assault, any pertinent comments or sensitive information ("I was raped") should be quoted directly and the source should be noted. Care should be taken to write clearly and spell correctly. Time should be documented for every intervention and reassessment. Any state or local reporting requirements must be met in documentation, and the contents of the prehospital report should remain confidential and be distributed only to appropriate healthcare providers. No data may be falsified, and any errors and steps taken to correct those errors must be documented.

DOCUMENTING PATIENT REFUSAL OF MEDICAL CARE

According to the Patient Self-Determination Act (1990), competent patients have the **right to refuse** any medical treatment, and parents have the right to make this decision for minor children. If a patient refuses care, then the EMS provider should inform the patient of the reasons to get medical care and possible consequences of refusal. The patient should be asked to sign the refusal form, and a family member, police officer, or bystander should sign as a witness to the patient's signing or witness the patient's refusal to sign. The EMS provider should complete documentation of any assessment carried out and any refusal of the patient to assessment. The provider should carefully document the conversation between the provider and patient regarding refusal of care and consequences and should document the proposed care as well as the information the provider gave the patient about alternate care (such as a visit to the personal physician) and the willingness to return if the patient has a change of mind.

SPECIAL DOCUMENTATION SITUATIONS

Additional documentation situations that should be handled according to protocol include:

- **Documentation errors**: In handwritten documents, draw one line through the error, initial, and write the correct information beside the error. If information was omitted, add a note with the date and initials. If documentation was electronic, follow the method prescribed for corrections.
- **Multiple-casualty incidents**: Record information temporarily for later complete documentation, if necessary, following the procedures in place for such an incident.
- **Incident reports**: Fill out forms as soon as possible, document any witnesses to the incident, and file forms according to protocol. Incident reports are often maintained separately from prehospital reports.
- **Special-situation reports**: Used for events/incidents that must be reported to an outside authority or as a supplement to the prehospital report. Fill out the report as soon as possible and include the names of all parties involved; use objective descriptions, and avoid stating conclusions. Maintain a personal copy.
- **Transfer reports**: Ensure that they contain minimum data sets and provide a transfer signature. These are used during hand-off.

EMS Communication

DYNAMICS OF THE COMMUNICATION PROCESS

The communication process, which includes the sender-receiver feedback loop, is based on Claude Shannon's article, "A Mathematical Theory of Communication" (1948), in which he provided the basis for information theory and described three necessary steps of successful communication: encoding a message, transmitting it through a channel, and decoding it. The resultant communication process begins with the sender, who serves as the encoder and determines the content of the message. The medium is the form the message takes (digital, written, audiovisual), and the channel is the method of delivery (mail, radio, TV, phone, email, text message). The recipient (receiver), who acts as the decoder, determines the meaning from the message. Feedback helps to determine whether or not the communication is successful and whether the message is understood as intended. This process is referred to as the sender-receiver feedback loop. Context is the environment (physical and psychological) in which the communication occurs, and interference is any factor that impacts the communication process. Interference may be external (such as environmental noise) or internal (such as emotional distress or anxiety).

EMS SYSTEM COMMUNICATION

With the **EMS personnel arrival** at the scene of an incident, he or she should assess the situation and the need for added resources, such as additional EMS personnel or police, and contact the appropriate authorities to request assistance. When additional EMS personnel arrive or contact is made with medical control or the receiving facility, the EMS provider should self-identify and provide a verbal report of the patient's current condition, including demographic information such as age and gender. The provider should report the patient's chief complaint and provide any history that is pertinent as well as the condition of the patient on arrival and any history of major illnesses. The EMS provider should also report the results of the patient assessment, including the vital signs and any physical/psychological findings, as well as any treatment provided and the patient's response to the treatment. The provider should communicate with law enforcement officers and other responders, such as firefighters, especially regarding safety concerns.

COMPONENTS

Components of an **EMS communication system** include the base station of a two-way radio system, which is in a fixed location, such as a dispatch center. The base station facilitates communication among a number of hand-held/mobile radios. There is often only one channel per base station, so additional base stations may be installed to add more channels. Radio transmitters/receivers may be vehicular mounted or mobile, although mobile transmitters/receivers may have limited range because they tend to have lower power (1–5 watts) than do base stations (20–50 watts). Typically, the mobile device has a range of 10–15 miles over average terrain, but it is shorter in rugged terrain. The Federal Communications Commission (FCC) controls radio frequencies, and those used for EMS are in the public safety pool.

COMMUNICATION WITH MEDICAL CONTROL

The EMS provider may be in communication with **medical control** regarding a patient's condition and need for medication. Medical control may be at the receiving facility or at a separate site. Upon receiving an order by phone or radio, the EMS provider should repeat back the order and dosage to ensure that the message was received correctly. When using the radio, the radio must be turned on and the press-to-talk (PTT) button must be pressed before beginning transmission. The provider should address the medical control person by name and give the name of their EMS unit. Transmissions should be brief and to the point, avoiding unnecessary pleasantries, codes, agency-specific terms, profanity, and meaningless phrases, keeping in mind that the airways are public. The

EMS provider should give individual digits for long numbers, use "affirmative" and "negative" in place of "yes" and "no," and say "over" when the transmission is finished. Reports should be objective rather than opinion based and should avoid offering a diagnosis. The dispatcher must be notified when the unit leaves the scene.

Phone/cellular communication is similar to radio communication, but EMS personnel should be familiar with important phone numbers (such as medical control, hospitals, trauma centers) or have the numbers prominently posted for access. They should also be aware of dead spots that may prevent communication and should have a backup plan (radio) for when cellular transmission fails.

EFFECTIVE COMMUNICATION AND INTERVIEW TECHNIQUES

Effective communication begins with a self-introduction and an introduction of other team members to the patient and family and includes respecting the patient's privacy by shielding the patient from passersby if possible and avoiding loudly repeating any patient information. If possible, the EMS provider should adjust lighting and limit outside distractions such as noise.

If possible, the patient should be **interviewed** alone or should be asked if he or she wants family members present. Verbal and nonverbal responses should be observed during an interview. Information should include not only the patient's facts but also the patient's attitude and concerns. The EMS provider should ask one question at a time in language that the patient understands and avoid providing false reassurances and advice or interrupting. Strategies include the following:

- Ask **open-ended informational questions** (as opposed to yes/no) with "who," "what," "where," "when," and "how," but avoid questions with "why" if possible.
    - Instead of "Why do you continue to use heroin?" ask "Have you tried to quit drug use?"
- Ask brief **clarifying questions**: "How long have you had weakness in your left side?"
- Provide a **list of options**: "Is your headache throbbing, stabbing, or dull?"
- **Rephrase/reflect** to encourage clarification.
    - Patient: "My husband had the same type of fall and died a month later."
    - EMS Provider: "You're afraid you might die from this fall."

SPECIAL INTERVIEW SITUATIONS

HOSTILE, AGGRESSIVE, OR IMPAIRED PATIENTS

Interviewing **hostile patients** requires a calm response, avoiding negative responses and using reflective statements, such as "I can understand your feelings." The EMS provider should maintain eye contact (50–60% of the time) and try to defuse the situation, but he or she should avoid staring or standing too close and having crossed arms because this may be misinterpreted as threatening behavior. If patients are **sexually aggressive**, it's important to tell them that the behavior is inappropriate and to ask them to stop. When interviewing patients under the **influence of drugs or alcohol**, try to ask essential questions such as the type and amount of drug/alcohol ingested. Obtain information from family or friends if necessary. When patients are **hearing impaired**, the EMS provider should face the person directly, speak slowly and distinctly (but avoid shouting), provide information in writing if possible, use pantomime, and try to reduce environmental noise. Knowledge of the alphabet in sign language can be very useful to communicate with the deaf, especially if a sign-language translator is unavailable.

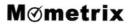

ELDERLY PATIENTS

When interviewing **elderly patients**, EMS personnel should be alert to possible cognitive, hearing, or vision impairments, especially if the patient appears confused upon questioning or his or her answers are inappropriate. They should ask if the patient has eyeglasses or a hearing aid and should obtain them if possible. The patient's family may be able to assist with the interview. If the patient's speech is unclear, he or she may need to put in dentures. When communicating with a **pediatric patient**, the EMS provider should have the parent or caregiver comfort the child and answer questions, especially if the child is an infant or is very young. The provider should use simple sentences and age-appropriate language and explain to the child what he or she is doing to help alleviate the child's fear. Adolescents should be addressed directly even if a parent or caregiver is providing some information, and, in some cases, the adolescent will provide more information if the parent/caregiver is not present.

NON-ENGLISH OR LIMITED ENGLISH-SPEAKING PATIENTS

The EMS provider should begin an interview with a **non-English or limited English-speaking patient** first in English. If a patient does not respond verbally and appears confused and/or frightened when questioned, and it is suspected that the patient doesn't speak English, the provider should ask directly if he or she can understand English. When a patient is a non-English speaking or a limited English speaker, the important thing is to communicate. Although children, friends, bystanders, and family are not usually used as translators, in emergent or life-threatening situations, an exception is made. The EMS provider may use signs, gestures, and pantomime to communicate and use simple words or phrases, such as "Pain?" and "OK?" because even non-English speakers may understand a few words. The provider may use a language line if available and the situation permits, and he or she should alert the receiving hospital of the need for a translator as well as providing information about the patient's language. The EMS provider should point to a body part before touching it.

THERAPEUTIC COMMUNICATION TECHNIQUES

Therapeutic communication begins with respect for the individual/family and the assumption that all communication, verbal and nonverbal, has meaning. Listening must be done empathetically. Techniques that facilitate communication include the following:

Introduction	Make a personal introduction and use the individual's name: "Mrs. Brown, I am Toby Williams, your EMS provider."
Encouragement	Use an open-ended opening question: "Is there anything you'd like to discuss?" Acknowledge comments: Say "yes" and "I understand." Allow silence and observe nonverbal behavior rather than trying to force a conversation. Ask for clarification if the patient's statements are unclear. Reflect the patient's statements back (use sparingly): • Individual: "I hate this hospital." • EMS Provider: "You hate this hospital?"
Empathy	Make observations: "You are shaking," and "You seem worried." Recognize feelings: • Individual: "I want to get well." • EMS Provider: "It must be hard for you to deal with this illness." Provide information as honestly and completely as possible about the patient's condition, treatment, and procedures and respond to the individual's questions and concerns.
Exploration	Verbally express implied messages: • Individual: "This treatment is too much trouble." • EMS Provider: "Do you think the treatment isn't helping you?" Explore a topic, but allow the individual to terminate the discussion without further probing: "I'd like to hear how you feel about that."
Orientation	Indicate reality: • Individual: "Someone is screaming." • EMS Provider: "That sound was a police siren." Comment on distortions without directly agreeing or disagreeing: • Individual: "That policeman promised I could go to St. John's Hospital." • EMS Provider: "Really? That's surprising because this ambulance is based at County Hospital."
Collaboration	Work together to achieve better results: "Maybe if we talk about this, we can figure out a way to make the treatment easier for you."
Validation	Seek validation: "Do you feel better now?" or "Did the medication help you breathe better?"

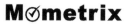

NONTHERAPEUTIC COMMUNICATION

Although using therapeutic communication is important, it is equally important to avoid interjecting **nontherapeutic communication**, which can effectively block effective communication. **Avoid the following**:

Stating meaningless clichés	"Don't worry. Everything will be fine." "Isn't it a nice day?"
Providing advice	"You should…" or "The best thing to do is…." It's better when individuals ask for advice to provide facts and encourage individuals to make their own decisions.
Providing inappropriate approval	This can prevent the individual from expressing true feelings or concerns. Individual: "I shouldn't cry about this." EMS Provider: "That's right. You're an adult."
Asking for explanations of behavior not directly related to individual care	Asking for explanations such as "Why are you upset?" may require analysis and an explanation of feelings on the individual's part.
Agreeing rather than accepting and responding	Agreeing with individual's statements "I agree with you" or "You are right" can make it difficult for the individual to change his/her statement or opinion later.
Making negative judgments	"You should stop arguing with the paramedics."
Devaluing an individual's feelings	"Everyone gets upset at times."
Disagreeing directly	"That can't be true" or "I think you are wrong."
Defending against criticism	"The doctor was not being rude; he's just very busy today."
Changing the subject	This avoids dealing with uncomfortable subjects: Individual: "I'm never going to get well." EMS Provider: "We'll contact your family in a few minutes."
Making inappropriate literal responses	Even as a joke, this is not appropriate, especially if the individual is confused or having difficulty expressing ideas: Individual: "There are bugs crawling under my skin." EMS Provider: "I'll get some bug spray."
Challenging to establish reality	This often increases confusion and frustration: Individual: "I'm dying!" EMS Provider: If you were dying, you wouldn't be able to yell and kick."
Filling silence with words	Some cultures and individuals allow more silent time in communication.

CULTURAL COMPETENCE

There are a number of issues related to cultural competence in communicating with others.

- **Eye contact:** Many cultures use eye contact differently than what is common in the United States. Some patients and families, such as Asians, Native Americans, and Arabs, may avoid direct eye contact, considering it rude, or they may look away to signal disapproval or may look down to signal respect. Careful observation of the way family members use eye contact can help to determine what will be most comfortable for the patient/family.
- **Distance**: Some cultures stand close to others (<4 feet) when speaking (Middle Easterners, Hispanics), and others stand at a greater distance (>4 feet) (Northern Europeans, many Americans). There is a considerable difference relating to concepts of personal space among cultures. Allowing the family to approach or observing whether they tend to move closer, lean forward, or move back can help to determine a comfortable distance for communication.
- **Time**: Americans tend to be time oriented, and they expect people to be on time, but time is viewed more flexibly in many other cultures.

CULTURAL CONSIDERATIONS

Cultural considerations when communicating with patients include the following:

Mexican

- Mexican culture perceives time with more flexibility than does American culture, so if patients/family need to be present at a particular time, the EMS provider should specify the exact time ("be here at 1:30 PM") and explain the reason rather than saying something that is more vague, such as "be here after lunch."
- People may appear to be unassertive or unable to make decisions when they are simply showing respect to the EMS provider by being deferent.
- In traditional families, the males make decisions, so a woman may wait for the husband or other males in the family to make decisions about her treatment or care.

Middle Eastern

- In Middle Eastern countries, males make the decisions, so issues for discussion or decision should be directed to males, such as the patient's spouse or son, and males may be direct in stating what they want, sometimes appearing demanding.
- Middle Easterners often require less personal space and may stand very close.
- If a male EMS provider must care for a female patient, then the family should be advised that *only* medical treatments, not personal care, will be done by the male provider.

Asian

- Asian families may expect EMS personnel to remain authoritative and to give directions and may not question their authority.
- Disagreeing is considered impolite. "Yes" may only mean that the person is heard, not that they agree with the person. When asked if they understand, they may indicate that they do even when they clearly do not so as not to offend the EMS provider.
- Asians may avoid eye contact as an indication of respect.

Legal and Ethical Issues

NEGLIGENCE

Negligence indicates that proper care has not been provided, based on established standards. Reasonable care uses a rationale for decision-making in relation to providing care. State regulations regarding negligence may vary, but they all have some statutes of limitation, governmental immunity, and Good Samaritan laws that may provide a defense. **Types of negligence** include:

- **Negligent conduct**: Failure to provide reasonable care or to protect/assist another, based on existing standards and expertise.
- **Gross negligence**: Willfully providing inadequate care while disregarding safety/security.
- **Contributory negligence**: The injured party contributes to his or her own harm.
- **Comparative negligence**: The amount of negligence attributed to each individual involved.

If the charge of negligence is supported, the patient may collect physical (lost earnings due to injury), psychological (pain and suffering), and punitive damages. The four necessary elements of negligence (failure to follow the standards of care) are as follows:

1. **Duty of care**: The defendant (healthcare provider) had a duty to provide adequate care and/or protect the plaintiff's (patient's) safety.
2. **Breach of duty**: The defendant failed to carry out the duty to care, resulting in danger, injury, or harm to the plaintiff.
3. **Damages**: The plaintiff experienced illness or injury as a result of the breach of duty.
4. **Causation**: The plaintiff's illness or injury is directly caused by the defendant's negligent breach of duty.

ADDITIONAL CIVIL AND CRIMINAL OFFENSES

Abandonment occurs if the EMS provider withdraws from providing care contrary to a patient's desire or knowledge and fails to arrange for appropriate care by others, resulting in harm to the patient. **Assault** occurs if an EMS provider threatens a patient in such a way that the patient becomes fearful of harm, whereas **battery** occurs when the EMS provider intentionally injures a patient, such as by hitting or shoving the person. Assault and battery often occur together.

STATUTORY RESPONSIBILITIES AND MANDATORY REPORTING

The EMS provider must practice within the **scope of responsibility**, which is outlined by each state's medical practice act. The EMS provider must be certified/licensed according to state requirements and meet appropriate educational standards regarding preparation and continuing education. The provider has a duty to the patients, the medical director, and the public and functions under government and medical oversight.

Although laws about **mandatory reporting** vary from state to state, healthcare providers, including EMS personnel, are considered mandatory reporters in all states and must report suspected cases of child and elder abuse and neglect. The EMS provider must follow state guidelines for reporting because simply notifying the receiving facility of suspected abuse or neglect is not adequate. The EMS provider should be familiar with the signs of abuse and neglect (certain types of fractures; unexplained or multiple bruises; suspicious bruise patterns; burns; hair loss; and inadequate food, clothing, and shelter).

EVIDENCE PRESERVATION

When an incident may involve **court cases**, such as with gunshot wounds, knife wounds, and rape, the EMS provider should take steps to **preserve evidence**, although providing emergent medical care takes priority. The provider should try to avoid disturbing items at the scene of the incident and should assess the environment and document any unusual findings, remembering that the environment and the patient are both considered to be part of the crime scene. The EMS provider should collaborate with law enforcement officers at the scene. If the patient has had a gunshot wound or a knife wound, the provider should not cut through the holes in the clothing but should cut along seams or away from the injuries. Any clothing or belongings removed during treatment should be secured separately in a paper bag (or plastic if paper is not available) and delivered with the patient to the receiving facility or to law enforcement officers. When the patient is describing the event, the EMS provider should document using quotations rather than summarizing.

ETHICS

ETHICAL PRINCIPLES AND MORAL OBLIGATIONS

Ethics is a branch of philosophy that studies morality—concepts of right and wrong. Applied ethics is the use of ethical principles, such as autonomy (right to self-determination), beneficence (acting to benefit another), nonmaleficence (doing no harm), verity (being truthful), and justice (equally distributing resources/care). Ethical conflicts may occur because of differences in cultural and ethical values, but they may also result from decisions that must be made regarding care, such as whether to provide CPR in a wilderness situation when the treatment is likely futile. They can also involve situations involving triage in which some patients are given priority over others, situations that involve professional misconduct (such as EMS personnel being abusive toward patients), and incidents of patient dumping because the patient has inadequate insurance or an inability to pay. EMS personnel have a moral obligation to make decisions about care in good faith and in the patient's best interest.

DECISION-MAKING MODELS

Decision-making models help guide the decision-making process on the basis of ethical principles:

- **Do no harm**: This model is based on nonmaleficence, the requirement that a treatment provided do no harm; however, by their nature, some treatments can and often do harm patients, so the underlying intent and goal of treatment must be considered when making decisions. For example, CPR may be carried out to save a patient's life and may be done with correct technique but still may result in rib fractures.
- **In good faith**: The motive for a decision should be honest and fair, and decisions should be made with a sincere intention to do good even though the outcome may be negative. For example, EMS personnel may provide a treatment for a patient in good faith although the treatment proves to be ineffective for that particular patient.
- **Patient's best interest**: Making a decision in the patient's best interest includes considering the patient's or parents' (in the case of children) wishes, the best clinical judgment, the best choice of various options, the chances for improvement/decline, and religious/cultural preferences.

Patient Rights

HEALTH INSURANCE PORTABILITY AND ACCOUNTABILITY ACT OF 1996 (HIPAA)

Sensitive information is classified under the **Health Insurance Portability and Accountability Act of 1996** (HIPAA) as protected health information (PHI) and includes the following:

- Any information about an individual's past, present, or future health or condition (mental or physical)
- Provision of health care
- Any identifying information related to payment for healthcare services, including name, address, Social Security number, or birth date, and any document or material that contains the identifying information

Personal information can be shared with a spouse, legal guardians, those with durable power of attorney for the patient, and those involved in the care of the patient, such as physicians, without a specific release. HIPAA mandates the following privacy and security rules to ensure that health information and individual privacy are protected:

- **Privacy rule**: Protected information includes any information included in the medical record (electronic or paper), conversations between the doctor and other healthcare providers, billing information, and any other form of health information.
- **Security rule**: Any electronic health information must be secure and protected against threats, hazards, or nonpermitted disclosure.

> **Review Video: HIPAA**
> Visit mometrix.com/academy and enter code: 412009

INFORMED CONSENT

Patients or their families must provide informed consent for all treatments that they receive. This includes a thorough explanation of all procedures, treatments, and associated risks. Patients/families should be apprised of all options and allowed input on the type of treatments. Patients/families should be apprised of all reasonable risks and any complications that might be life threatening or increase morbidity.

The American Medical Association has established **guidelines for informed consent**. Informed consent includes all of the following components:

- Explanation of the diagnosis
- Nature of and reason for the treatment or procedure
- Risks and benefits
- Alternative options (regardless of cost or insurance coverage)
- Risks and benefits of alternative options
- Risks and benefits of not having a treatment or procedure

Obtaining informed consent is a requirement in all states. The requirement for informed consent may be waived in life-threatening situations and if the EMS provider cannot obtain informed consent because the patient cannot communicate and legal consent cannot be obtained.

CONDITIONS FOR CONSENT

The conditions for consent for care and decision-making capacity include the following:

- **18 years or older OR court-emancipated minors**: Patients who are younger (and not court-emancipated) may have the right to give consent for all or some medical treatment in some states. State laws vary; for example, the age of consent for medical treatment in Alabama is 14.
- **Mentally competent to make decisions**: Impairment by mental disability, injury, illness, or substance abuse (intoxication) may impede an adult's ability to provide consent.

Consent may be expressed if the patient is able to give informed consent, or it may be implied, such as when care is provided in an emergent situation in which the patient is unable to give consent. Parents or caregivers give consent for minors younger than the age of 18 unless they have been emancipated. If parents or caregivers are unavailable to give consent, life-saving emergent care, general medical assessment, and medical care to prevent further injury or harm can be provided without consent.

ADVANCE DIRECTIVES, DURABLE POWER OF ATTORNEY, AND DO-NOT-RESUSCITATE (DNR) ORDER

In accordance with federal and state laws, individuals have the **right to self-determination** in health care, including decisions about end-of-life care through **advance directives** such as living wills and the right to assign a surrogate person to make decisions through a **durable power of attorney**. Patients should routinely be questioned about an advanced directive because they may present at a healthcare organization without the document. Patients who have indicated that they desire a **do-not-resuscitate (DNR) order** should not receive resuscitative treatments for terminal illness or conditions in which meaningful recovery cannot occur. Patients and families of those with terminal illnesses should be questioned as to whether the patients are hospice patients. For those with DNR requests or those withdrawing life support, staff should provide the patient palliative rather than curative measures, such as pain control and/or oxygen, and emotional support to the patient and family. Religious traditions and beliefs about death should be treated with respect.

HUMAN RESEARCH SUBJECT PROTECTION

Protection of human subjects is covered in the Health and Human Services, Title 45 Code of Federal Regulations, part 46. This regulation provides guidance for institutional review boards (IRBs) for those involved in research and outlines requirements. Institutions engaged in nonexempt research must submit an assurance of compliance (document) to the **Office for Human Research Protections** (OHRP), agreeing to comply with all requirements for research projects. Subjects cannot be used solely as a means to an end, but research should hold the possibility of benefit to the subject. Risks should be minimal, and selection of subjects should be equitable. Some research populations are granted additional protections because of their vulnerability and susceptibility to coercion; these populations include children, prisoners, pregnant women, human fetuses and neonates, mentally disabled people, and people who are economically or educationally disadvantaged. When cooperative research projects are conducted involving more than one institution, then each must safeguard the rights of subjects, ensuring informed consent and privacy.

Abuse and Neglect

ELDER ABUSE

Types of elder abuse include the following:

- **Physical**: Various types of assault related to hitting, kicking, pulling hair, shoving, and pushing. Patients may be forcibly confined, forced into seclusion, and/or force-fed to the point that they choke on food.
- **Psychological**: Caregivers may threaten to hit the patient, brandish a weapon, and/or tell the person to commit suicide. Ongoing intimidation may make the patient terrified and anxious. Sometimes, caregivers threaten to injure pets or family members, increasing the patient's fear.
- **Sexual**: Types of sexual abuse include the following:
  - Physical: Fondling, kissing, and rape
  - Emotional: Exhibitionism
  - Verbal: Sexual harassment, using obscene language, and threatening
- **Financial**: Financial abuse includes the following:
  - Outright stealing of property or persuading patients to give away possessions
  - Forcing patients to sign away property
  - Emptying bank and savings accounts and using stolen credit cards
  - Convincing the person to invest money in fraudulent schemes
  - Taking money for home renovations that are not done

CHILD ABUSE

Children rarely admit to abuse (physical, sexual, or emotional) and often attempt to protect the abusing parent. Therefore, suspicion of abuse depends on other indicators such as the following:

- **Behavioral**: The child may be overly compliant or fearful with obvious changes in demeanor when a parent/caregiver is present. Some children act out with aggression toward other children or animals. Children may become depressed, suicidal, or present with sleeping or eating disorders. Behaviors may become increasingly self-destructive as the child ages, including inappropriate sexualized behavior.
- **Physical/Sexual**: The type, location, and extent of injuries can raise the suspicion of abuse. Head and facial injuries and bruising are common signs of physical abuse, as are bite or burn marks and spiral fractures. There may be handprints or grab marks and unusual bruising, such as across the buttocks. Any bruising, swelling, or tearing of the genital area and the identification of sexually transmitted infections are also causes for concern.

Suspected abuse must be reported to the appropriate authorities, according to protocol, with careful documentation of findings and statements by the child or caregivers.

INJURIES CONSISTENT WITH DOMESTIC VIOLENCE/ABUSE

Injuries consistent with domestic violence/abuse include the following:

- Characteristic injuries:
  - Ruptured eardrum
  - Rectal/genital injury—burns, bites, trauma
  - Scrapes and bruises about the neck, face, head, trunk, arms
  - Cuts, bruises, and fractures of the face
- Patterns of injuries:
  - "Bathing suit" pattern—injuries on parts of body that are usually covered with clothing because the perpetrator wants to hide the evidence of abuse
  - Head and neck injuries (50%)
- Abusive injuries (rarely attributable to accidents):
  - Bites, bruises, rope and cigarette burns, and welts in the outline of weapons (belt marks)
  - Bilateral injuries of the arms/legs
- Defensive injuries:
  - Back-of-the-body injury from being attacked while crouched on the floor facedown
  - Located on the soles of the feet from kicking at a perpetrator
  - Located on the ulnar aspect of the hands or palm from blocking blows

NEGLECT AND LACK OF SUPERVISED CARE

Children and older or impaired adults may suffer from profound **neglect or a lack of supervision** that places them at risk. Indicators include the following:

- Appearing dirty and unkempt, sometimes with infestations of lice, and wearing ill-fitting, torn clothing and shoes.
- Being tired and sleepy during the daytime.
- Having excessive medical or dental problems, such as extensive dental caries.
- Missing doctor appointments and not receiving proper immunizations.
- Being underweight for their current stage of development.
- Lacking assistive devices or misplaced hearing aids/eyeglasses.
- Left in soiled or urine-/feces-soiled clothing.
- Clothing is inadequate (such as lack of a coat/sweater during winter or dirty, torn, ill-fitting clothes).

Neglect can be difficult to assess, especially if the EMS provider is serving a homeless or very disadvantaged population. Home visits may be needed to ascertain if there is adequate food, clothing, or supervision, and this is beyond the scope of care provided by the EMS provider. Thus, suspicions should be reported to the appropriate authorities who can arrange a follow-up assessment of the home environment.

Public Health

PUBLIC HEALTH SYSTEM

EMS are part of the **public health system**, a network of private, nonprofit, and government agencies and healthcare providers providing public health services in a wide range of areas. The primary services provided by the public health system include the following:

- Monitoring community health
- Identifying hazards to health in the environment and the community
- Educating people about health issues
- Mobilizing various agencies and individuals to take action
- Enforcing public safety laws and regulations
- Ensuring that healthcare providers are qualified, licensed, and certified as required
- Ensuring that health care is available
- Assessing the effectiveness of health care
- Researching health problems and finding solutions

Public health laws and regulations may be federal, state, or tribal and may cover issues such as immunization requirements, drinking water and sewage system standards, air quality, water fluoridation, restrictions on tobacco use (age and place), restrictions on drinking (age, driving), speed limits, prenatal care, abuse (child, older adult, sexual, and domestic), safety equipment, and safe lifting. Healthy People 2030, from the U.S. Department of Health and Human Services, provides goals and objectives for health-related public policies.

PUBLIC EDUCATION REGARDING SAFETY MEASURES

EMS personnel are often involved in **public education** regarding the following safety measures:

- **Car seats**: Car seats should be properly secured in the backseat of a motor vehicle. They should be rear facing for infants and toddlers up to 2 years of age (or the maximum recommended height and weight) and forward-facing with a harness for toddlers and preschoolers. School-aged children should use booster seats with a belt and harness until they are at least 4 feet 9 inches tall. Children younger than age 13 should not ride in a front seat.
- **Seat belts**: All people in a motor vehicle should be secured with seat belts and shoulder harnesses.
- **Helmets**: Helmets should fit properly and snugly, cover the top of the forehead, and have a securing chinstrap. They should be worn when riding a bicycle or motorcycle and engaging in sports activities such as rollerblading but not on playground equipment or when climbing trees.

Additional safety equipment that EMS personnel should be familiar with includes home alarms (smoke alarms and carbon monoxide alarms) and mobility aids for fall prevention such as safety rails, grab bars, canes, and walkers.

LEVELS OF DISEASE PREVENTION

Levels of disease prevention include the following:

- **Primary**: The goal is to prevent the initial occurrence of a health problem, such as a disease or injury, through activities such as immunizations, smoking cessation, fluoride supplementation of water, promotion of seat belt and helmet use, and use of child car seat restraints. Interventions are often aimed at the general public or large groups of people.
- **Secondary**: The goal is to identify diseases or conditions quickly and provide prompt intervention to provide treatment and prevent further disability through activities such as BP screenings, breast and testicular self-examinations, hearing and vision screenings, mammography, and pregnancy testing.
- **Tertiary**: The goal is to assist those who already have disease or disability to prevent further progress of the disease and to allow people to achieve the maximum quality of life through activities such as support groups, counseling, diet and exercise, stress management, and supportive services.

EMT Practice Test #1

1. What does proper treatment of a hostile or aggressive patient include?

- a. Restraining the patient
- b. Encouraging the patient to accept emergency care
- c. Calling a physician
- d. Watching for sudden changes in behavior

2. What should you do in the case of a patient with gastric distention and vomiting?

- a. Turn the patient's head.
- b. Roll the patient onto his or her side.
- c. Place the patient in a supine position.
- d. Perform rescue breathing.

3. According to HIPAA regulations, protected patient information is information that relates to any of the following EXCEPT?

- a. Medical conditions.
- b. Hospital billing information.
- c. Medical care.
- d. School records.

4. Which of the following is the correct sequence of connective function?

- a. Muscle-ligament-bone
- b. Bone-muscle-ligament
- c. Muscle-tendon-bone
- d. Muscle-bone-tendon

5. You are providing emergency care to a hypothermic patient. All of the following are appropriate treatment steps EXCEPT:

- a. Allow the patient to walk to a warmer place
- b. Cover the patient with as many blankets as are available
- c. Utilize heat packs wrapped in towels around the armpits, neck, head, and groin areas
- d. Provide warm, humidified oxygen

6. Which of the following statements is NOT true regarding the use of a tourniquet?

- a. The tourniquet is considered to be a last-resort way to treat bleeding.
- b. A tourniquet should be placed directly over a joint to maximize its effectiveness.
- c. Once a tourniquet is applied, it should not be taken off, because it may cause blood clots to mobilize.
- d. The tourniquet should be plainly visible, so anyone else who comes to treat the patient will easily see it.

7. What is the main mechanism of action for activated charcoal?

- a. It induces vomiting.
- b. It intravenously binds the toxin as it is absorbed to prevent side effects.
- c. It binds the toxin in the gut to prevent absorption.
- d. It neutralizes acid- or alkali-type toxic substances in the gut.

189

8. A diving injury is likely to cause which of the following injuries?

    a. Distraction injury
    b. Whiplash
    c. Compression injury
    d. Lateral bending injury

9. How long is the average length of a woman's first labor?

    a. 10 to 12 hours
    b. 12 to 18 hours
    c. 18 to 20 hours
    d. 18 to 24 hours

10. In treating an ankle or foot injury, what should you do?

    a. Apply manual traction.
    b. Apply an ice pack directly to the skin.
    c. Change the position of the ankle.
    d. Tie a pillow to the ankle and foot.

11. During your initial assessment of a patient, your general impression takes only a few seconds. While forming your general impression, what is the most important goal?

    a. Diagnose the patient's illness and note the age, gender, and race.
    b. Prioritize care, form a plan of action, and establish nature of illness or mechanism of injury.
    c. Determine if there are life-threatening injuries.
    d. Transport the patient, provide oxygen if needed, and start IV therapy.

12. Which of the following would be the most appropriate choice for positioning an unresponsive patient with suspected trauma in order to open the airway?

    a. Jaw thrust technique
    b. Head-tilt chin-lift technique
    c. Triple-airway maneuver
    d. Side-facing chin-lift technique

13. Which of the following individuals is least likely to give expressed consent?

    a. A 30-year-old who is legal guardian for a 10-year-old child
    b. A 45-year-old man with a blood alcohol level of over twice the legal limit
    c. A young woman who recently celebrated her 18th birthday
    d. A 75-year-old man with cancer and a do-not-resuscitate order

14. A woman in her 34th week of pregnancy presents with vaginal bleeding. From your EMT training, you know this type of bleeding is likely indicative of which of the following?

    a. An issue with the placenta
    b. Premature delivery
    c. Impending miscarriage
    d. Preeclampsia

15. When the heart does not receive adequate oxygen, the patient may feel pain in the chest, especially following exertion. What is the medical term for this type of pain?

a. Angina
b. Dyspnea
c. Congestive heart failure
d. Tachycardia

16. Which of the following terms refers to a condition in which the heart is "quivering" and not producing a pulse?

a. Ventricular tachycardia
b. Atrial tachycardia
c. Heart block
d. Fibrillation

17. Which of the following situations requires the use of the automatic external defibrillator (AED)?

a. You are unable to hear the heartbeat, although you can feel a weak carotid pulse.
b. You are unable to hear the heartbeat, and unable to palpate any pulse.
c. The patient is awake but has a very irregular heart rhythm.
d. The patient is unresponsive, but you note a pedal pulse.

18. What color is amniotic fluid normally?

a. Greenish
b. Brownish
c. Clear
d. Mixed with blood

19. Which of the following is an example of what you would NOT do if you suspect a three-year-old child has a foreign body airway obstruction according to AHA guidelines?

a. Visualize the airway and remove the foreign object using a finger sweep if you are able.
b. Perform back blows.
c. Perform abdominal thrusts.
d. If the child is not breathing and is unresponsive, give two breaths, then look for a foreign body in the airway.

20. You make an error while writing your report of patient care. What is the correct method of correcting the mistake?

a. Erase and enter the information correctly.
b. Obliterate it completely with heavy pen marks, and then rewrite it.
c. Simply white it out with correction fluid, and then rewrite it.
d. Strike through the error with one horizontal line, and then initial and rewrite it.

21. What is the correct position for releasing chest compression?

a. With elbows locked, remove pressure from the patient's chest by lifting at the hips, while maintaining light contact.
b. Lift the hands away from the patient's chest by bending at the elbows.
c. Remove full contact from the chest and by straightening back.
d. Keep knees, back, and elbows bent to allow for full recoil while minimizing time without contact on the patient.

22. What should you do if an adult patient has stopped breathing but has a pulse?

a. Perform chest compressions.
b. Initiate CPR.
c. Provide rescue breaths.
d. Use the finger to do a blind sweep of the mouth to remove any foreign objects.

23. Which of the following is NOT meant by the abbreviation AOx3?

a. The patient is oriented to the time.
b. The patient is oriented to his person.
c. The patient is oriented to the place.
d. The patient is ambulatory.

24. All of the following are layers of the skin EXCEPT:

a. Epidermis
b. Sebaceous
c. Dermis
d. Subcutaneous

25. All of the following are immobilization devices used for spine or neck injuries EXCEPT:

a. Cervical collar
b. Long spine board
c. Short backboard
d. Thoracolumbar orthosis

26. You are responding to a patient in the field with respiratory arrest with a trained paramedic. The paramedic has successfully placed an endotracheal tube and confirmed placement with different techniques. The patient is now stable and ready to be transported to the hospital. You assist to load the patient onto the ambulance. As you begin to head to the hospital, the patient's oxygen saturation level begins to drop as well as the heart rate. What should you immediately suspect is the issue?

a. The patient has gone into cardiac arrest.
b. The endotracheal tube has dislodged and is no longer in the proper position.
c. The patient possibly has pneumonia.
d. The patient has gone into shock.

27. Which primary intervention gives the patient the greatest chance for survival of a cardiac arrest?

a. IV therapy
b. Nitroglycerin
c. Defibrillation
d. Oxygen administration

28. When using directional terminology to describe an injury that is on an extremity, near the trunk, what is the best term?

a. Distal
b. Proximal
c. Posterior
d. Lateral

29. You arrive on the scene following a call for respiratory distress. The patient appears to be thin, barrel-chested, and breathing through pursed lips. You notice an oxygen tank nearby. What is your immediate assessment?

   a. Emphysema
   b. Chronic bronchitis
   c. Asthma
   d. Pneumonia

30. Which type of poisoning may require the administration of activated charcoal?

   a. Ingested poison
   b. Absorbed poison
   c. Injected poison
   d. Inhaled poison

31. Which of the following is the most important statement about treating patients with respiratory distress?

   a. Oxygen should be administered immediately.
   b. A spacer should always be used with inhalers.
   c. Medical authorization should be obtained before administering an inhaler.
   d. Immediately begin the focused history and physical in order to determine what you are dealing with.

32. Which of the following set of baseline vital signs would be most concerning to you?

   a. A 12-year-old boy with a pulse of 110, respiratory rate of 20, and blood pressure of 95/60
   b. A newborn baby with a pulse of 155, respiratory rate of 52, and blood pressure of 85/40
   c. A 3-year-old girl with a pulse of 80, respiratory rate of 30, and blood pressure of 82/45
   d. A 16-year-old boy with a pulse of 100, respiratory rate of 25, and blood pressure of 100/60

33. What is the name of the document that explains the type of chemical and first-aid care for that chemical exposure?

   a. Chemical information sheet (CIS)
   b. *Physicians' Desk Reference* (PDR)
   c. Safety data sheet (SDS)
   d. Poison control data (PCD)

34. Which of the following statements is inaccurate regarding the administration of oral glucose gel?

   a. Place the tip of the tube between the cheek and the gum.
   b. If the patient is unconscious, administer the gel very slowly.
   c. Do not administer oral glucose to any patient that is vomiting.
   d. Perform ongoing assessments every five minutes until the patient is stable.

35. What is a dangerous pulse rate for an adult in an emergency situation?

   a. Above 100 beats per minute
   b. Below 50 beats per minute
   c. 60 beats per minute
   d. 90 beats per minute

36. What is the name of the disease that causes thinning of the bones and loss of bone density?

    a. Osteogenesis imperfecta
    b. Osteoporosis
    c. Paget's disease
    d. Osteosarcoma

37. A hip fracture is a fracture of which of the following?

    a. Pelvis
    b. Proximal femur
    c. Pubic bone
    d. Humerus bone

38. A patient is in full respiratory arrest and will likely not survive the arrest. The EMT learns the patient is an organ donor. What is the appropriate way to proceed?

    a. Continue to provide treatment at an appropriate level based on the patient's condition.
    b. Immediately stop care and provide comfort to the patient.
    c. Contact the patient's family to pay their last respects.
    d. Contact the medical director for advice on how to proceed.

39. Which of the following is a sign of iron poisoning in a child?

    a. Hyperventilation
    b. Drowsiness
    c. Irritability
    d. Bloody vomiting

Refer to the following for questions 40-42:

> You receive a call from a panicked taxicab driver, telling you that a woman is having a baby in his cab. When you arrive, a crowd has gathered around the cab. A woman is lying in the back seat, moaning. She complains of needing to go to the bathroom.

40. What is the first step in caring for this patient?

    a. Allow her to go to the bathroom.
    b. Tell bystanders to leave.
    c. Transport the patient to the hospital.
    d. Remove the patient's clothing to view the vaginal opening.

41. Bulging is visible at the vaginal opening. The patient insists that she does not want to have the baby in the cab and begs you to take her to the hospital. What should you do?

    a. Transport the patient to the hospital.
    b. Elevate the patient's buttocks with blankets or a pillow and prepare for delivery.
    c. Prepare for delivery by positioning the patient with one foot on the car seat and one on the floor.
    d. Time the patient's contractions.

42. In delivering the baby, what should you do?
a. Place one hand below the baby's head.
b. Gently pull on the baby to facilitate delivery.
c. Once the head delivers, tell the mother to push.
d. Gently grasp the baby by the feet.

43. What is the term that is used for hypoperfusion resulting from the massive loss of blood?
a. Hypovolemic shock
b. Hemorrhagic shock
c. Cardiogenic shock
d. Electrical shock

44. What should you do in the care of a patient with hazardous materials injuries?
a. Make sure the patient has been decontaminated.
b. Transport the patient immediately.
c. Begin care only after the patient has been moved to a safe zone.
d. Wait for arrival of the hazardous materials (hazmat) team before treating the patient.

45. What does emergency care for a snakebite include?
a. Cleaning the bite with soap and water
b. Placing ice on the bite
c. Sucking the venom from the bite
d. Capturing the snake

46. A child with developmental delays has a tracheostomy tube inserted to help him breathe at home. The tracheostomy tube has become dislodged, and the parents have not been able to replace it. The child is going into respiratory distress. What should you do before the patient is transported?
a. Try to relodge the tracheostomy.
b. Perform CPR.
c. Cover the stoma and ventilate with a bag-valve-mask over the mouth and nose.
d. Ventilate through the stoma with a bag-valve-mask.

47. Which of the following is the most significant sign of hypoperfusion during an allergic reaction?
a. Rash
b. Edema
c. Altered mental state
d. Wheezing

48. You arrive at a multiple vehicle accident where a nonbreathing patient appears to have a cervical spine injury. What do you do to modify your ventilation technique?
a. Have a second EMT stabilize the patient's head or use your knees to prevent movement.
b. Use the head tilt to open the airway.
c. Push down on the chin to open the airway.
d. Position yourself over the patient's chest to best observe the respirations.

Refer to the following for questions 49-51:

> The morning after a snow storm, the ski patrol discovers the wreckage of an automobile on the road to a ski lodge. A 70-year-old man is trapped inside. He is disoriented but conscious and has suffered a broken hip. He exhibits severe muscular rigidity and has no memory of the events before or after the accident. The patient's wife had reported the man missing the previous night after he became intoxicated and was ejected from a local bar.

49. In addition to a broken hip, what else is this patient is suffering from?

    a. Hypoperfusion
    b. Inadequate circulation
    c. Hypothermia
    d. Psychiatric disorder

50. What should you do to prevent heat loss in an injured patient?

    a. Perform active rewarming techniques.
    b. Massage the extremities.
    c. Administer a stimulant.
    d. Use blankets to provide a barrier to the outside.

51. What is body heat loss often associated with?

    a. Alcohol intoxication
    b. Head trauma
    c. Cardiac events
    d. Altered mental status

52. In order for an EMT to be considered negligent, four criteria must be met. Which of the following is NOT considered one of the criteria?

    a. The EMT failed to provide emergency services.
    b. The injury to the patient was directly caused by the omission of a specific treatment that would have helped the patient.
    c. Due to an EMT's inability to make it through traffic, emergency medical treatment was delayed and patient death occurred.
    d. The EMT failed to provide the appropriate level of service that another EMT with similar education, training, and experience would have provided in the same type of case.

53. The average pulse for a five-year-old falls within what range?

    a. 70 to 115
    b. 60 to 80
    c. 100 to 140
    d. 50 to 70

54. In removing an injured child from a car safety seat, what should you do?

    a. Slide the child out of the seat.
    b. Strap the child across the abdomen.
    c. Tape the child across the chin.
    d. Apply a cervical collar.

55. You arrive on the scene to find an 80-year-old man in full cardiac arrest. The man's daughter tells you that he has a DNR order, but she is unable to provide verification of this. What should you do?

   a. Provide comfort care and transport the patient to the hospital to verify the DNR order.
   b. Begin CPR, because written documentation is required for a DNR order.
   c. Attempt to contact the patient's primary care physician.
   d. Try to contact other family members to verify the DNR order.

56. In providing emergency care for a patient with shock, after putting on appropriate bodily substance precautions, what are most important steps to follow next?

   a. Stop the bleeding and prevent heat loss.
   b. Assess the airway/ventilate and stop the bleeding.
   c. Assess the airway/ventilate and prevent heat loss.
   d. Stop the bleeding and transport immediately.

57. What is the name for a closed injury in which there is cellular damage under the dermis with discoloration?

   a. Burn
   b. TBI
   c. Concussion
   d. Contusion

58. You have intubated a patient and need to check placement of the endotracheal tube. Breath sounds are not audible in the area of the lungs, but you do hear a gurgling sound. How do you interpret this type of noise?

   a. The endotracheal tube is in the proper position.
   b. The endotracheal tube is almost in the correct position, but it needs to be advanced a few millimeters more.
   c. The endotracheal tube is located in the esophagus.
   d. The endotracheal tube needs to be pulled back by a few millimeters.

59. You arrive at a multiple-vehicle accident and prepare to transport an injured patient who states that he cannot feel his legs. Upon examination of his lower extremities, you notice that both legs appear to have dilated veins. What do you suspect?

   a. Anaphylactic shock
   b. Septic shock
   c. Hypovolemic shock
   d. Neurogenic shock

Refer to the following for questions 60-62:

> A 38-year-old woman falls through the ice while skating on a frozen pond with her 6-year-old daughter. While the child went to get help, her mother remained trapped waist-deep in the freezing water for several hours. After rescue, the woman reports that her toes are freezing. On assessment, her toes appear grayish-blue in color and feel frozen to the touch.

60. **What would be the first step in caring for this patient?**
    a. Squeeze the toes to increase circulation.
    b. Perform active rewarming.
    c. Massage the toes to increase circulation.
    d. Administer high-concentration oxygen.

61. **Transport to the hospital has been severely delayed due to icy road conditions. A rescue worker offers the patient a drink of an alcoholic beverage from a flask to keep her warm. What is the next step in treating this patient?**
    a. Continue to massage the frozen area.
    b. Begin active rewarming.
    c. Heat a container of water and immerse the patient's feet until they touch the bottom.
    d. Keep the frozen area covered and allow the patient to sip the alcoholic beverage.

62. **All of the following are true of active external rewarming EXCEPT:**
    a. Warm water bottles can be applied to the groin and axilla.
    b. Warm blankets or forced air systems such as the Bair Hugger are appropriate.
    c. There is little evidence supporting active external rewarming being effective in the context of moderate to severe hypothermia.
    d. There are risks for rebound hypothermia after the warming is discontinued.

63. **What is the preferred method for moving a patient down a set of stairs?**
    a. Carry the patient on your back.
    b. Use a stair chair.
    c. Carry the patient on a stretcher.
    d. Lean forward from your hips.

64. **What is the preferred method of ventilation in the field for a patient who is not able to breathe on his or her own?**
    a. Mouth-to-mouth ventilation
    b. Mouth-to-mask ventilation
    c. Two-person bag-valve-mask
    d. One-person bag-valve-mask

65. **Why is it important for a patient in shock to remain warm?**
    a. To prevent oxygen from being wasted as shivering occurs
    b. The patient will respond better to treatment if warm
    c. To help maintain blood pressure
    d. To keep the patient comfortable

66. **What is a potentially serious sign or symptom associated with an acute stress reaction?**
    a. Difficulty sleeping
    b. Nausea
    c. Loss of appetite
    d. Uncontrollable crying

67. When a patient experiences stabbing chest pain that increases in severity when taking a deep breath, what is the probable origin of the discomfort?

    a. Circulatory system
    b. GI tract
    c. Gallbladder
    d. Respiratory system

68. What is the proper order for securing the straps on the KED?

    a. Head, top, middle, bottom, legs
    b. Head, legs, top, middle, bottom
    c. Legs, head, top, bottom, middle
    d. Middle, bottom, legs, head, top

69. What is the medical terminology for breathing too fast and shallow?

    a. Bradypnea
    b. Dyspnea
    c. Tachypnea
    d. Bronchiectasis

70. When inserting a nasopharyngeal airway, what technique is appropriate?

    a. The correct-size airway would extend from the tip of the nose to the larynx.
    b. Insert the airway through the narrowest nostril.
    c. Insert the airway with the bevel up.
    d. Use a water-soluble lubricant.

71. While off duty, you observe a severe car accident, with one of the vehicles overturned. What should your procedure include?

    a. Provide care to the victims, then leave the scene.
    b. Provide care and wait for additional help to arrive.
    c. Call 911 and leave the scene.
    d. Begin care, call for additional help, then leave the scene.

Refer to the following for questions 72-74:

> You and your partner are called to the home of a 75-year-old man complaining of severe pain in the chest and nausea. As the patient is being assessed, he suddenly loses consciousness.

72. What is the first step in treating a patient with severe chest pain?

    a. Obtain a patient history.
    b. Administer oxygen.
    c. Perform a physical exam.
    d. Obtain baseline vital signs.

73. What is the first step in treating a patient who loses consciousness?

    a. Obtain a pulse.
    b. Assess breathing.
    c. Attach an automated external defibrillator.
    d. Open the airway.

74. What is the best way to decrease oxygen demand in the case of cardiac compromise?
   a. Transport the patient immediately, flashing lights, and using the siren.
   b. Reassure the patient.
   c. Travel at high speeds but without the siren.
   d. Give the patient nitroglycerin.

75. If a child is afraid of having an oxygen mask placed directly on their face, what is an alternate method?
   a. Nasal airway
   b. Endotracheal tube
   c. Oral airway
   d. Blow-by oxygen

76. As you are assessing an infant's APGAR scores, you realize that the infant's heart rate is 78 beats per minute. What should you do next?
   a. Provide artificial ventilations at a rate of 15 liters per minute and reassess after 30 seconds.
   b. Provide positive pressure ventilations at a rate of 30 to 60 per minute and reassess after 30 seconds.
   c. Start chest compressions according to newborn standards and reassess in 1 minute. If the heart rate is above 100 beats per minute, stop the compressions and administer high-flow oxygen via a nonrebreather mask.
   d. Provide oxygen, initiate cardiac monitoring with a 12-lead EKG, and continue to monitor the patient's status.

77. What is the medical term that describes a patient who is responding inappropriately, either verbally or nonverbally?
   a. Altered mental status
   b. Seizure
   c. Coma
   d. Hypoglycemia

78. What is the term for the stage of labor in which the head of the baby is bulging from the vaginal orifice?
   a. Crowning
   b. Pushing
   c. Bloody show
   d. Dilation

Answer Key and Explanations for Test #1

1. D: The best approach in treating a hostile or aggressive patient is to watch for sudden changes in behavior and seek assistance from law enforcement. Restraining the patient or forcing him or her to accept emergency care is usually not in the legal jurisdiction of an EMT.

2. B: Rescue breathing can blow air into the patient's stomach, causing distention. In the case of gastric distention and vomiting, roll the patient onto his or her side. Simply turning the patient's head can lead to aspiration of vomitus or aggravation of spinal injury.

3. D: HIPAA regulations define protected patient information as anything related to medical care, hospital billing, or medical diagnoses. This information cannot be disclosed without proper consent being obtained or without information being deidentified. HIPAA regulations do not apply to schools, and therefore school records are not subject to HIPAA's privacy laws.

4. C: The correct sequence of connective function is muscle-tendon-bone and bone-ligament-bone.

5. A: There are three stages of hypothermia. First the patient is alert and oriented, second the patient is becoming disoriented and unresponsive, and third the patient is unresponsive. Vital signs begin to change drastically as the body tries to adapt to declining body temperature. Hypothermic patients may act like they are drunk, and in fact, alcohol can worsen the effects of hypothermia. The patient's ability to make decisions may be clouded by both the hypothermia as well as alcohol. The main goal of treatment is to begin to raise the body temperature. This can be done by covering the patient with blankets and placing heat packs warmed to a temperature of 102–104 °F at strategic places around the body. Oxygen should ideally be administered in a humidified, warm form. These warming steps will not cure the patient but will prevent further heat loss from occurring. The patient should not be allowed to walk because of the possibility of irregular heart rhythms that could potentially be fatal.

6. B: The use of a tourniquet is considered a last resort when other methods for controlling bleeding have failed. Using a tourniquet often will cause permanent and serious damage to surrounding muscles, tissue, nerves, and blood vessels. The majority of the time, amputation will result if a tourniquet is used. If the decision to use a tourniquet has been carefully made, a wide tourniquet should be used instead of an item such as a belt, piece of rope, or a wire. The key is to provide continuous pressure around the entire perimeter of the injury. It should not be placed directly on a joint but rather as close to the bleeding site as is possible. It is imperative that the tourniquet not be removed after it has been applied because blood clots could potentially mobilize and head to the lungs, causing a pulmonary embolism and possibly death. The use of the tourniquet should be documented carefully and communicated with anyone who may be caring for the patient.

7. C: Activated charcoal is one of the main interventions for the management of poison ingestion. The trade names include Actidose, Liqui-Char, and Insta-Char. Activated charcoal is orally administered under medical direction. The mechanism of action is to bind the toxin or poison in the stomach to prevent absorption from occurring. It only works on ingested toxins and not inhaled, injected, or other routes. Activated charcoal should not be used if a patient has ingested either an acid or an alkali substance. It should also be avoided in patients who are unable to swallow or who have a decreased mental status. If a patient receives the activated charcoal early in the course, the outcome is significantly improved. Activated charcoal may cause vomiting, and the dose may need to be given again for optimal effectiveness. The adult dose is usually 25 to 50 grams, while the dose for a child is 12.5 to 25 grams.

8. C: As the EMS team approaches the scene of an accident, it should be quickly assessed for types of possible injuries. In the case of a diving accident, compression injury to the spine is likely, but it can also occur in motor vehicle accidents and falls. A distraction injury is tearing or stretching of the spinal cord and occurs in hanging situations as well as gunshot wounds to the spinal cord area. Lateral bending injuries are where the head and neck are bent too far to the side beyond what the body is normally capable of. This is also known as whiplash and can occur in motor vehicle accidents where the car was hit from behind. Stabilization and immobilization are key to initiating treatment in these types of cases.

9. B: The average length of labor for first-time mothers is 12 to 18 hours. This can vary widely though and is unique to each mother. The length of labor tends to decrease with each subsequent baby. Questions need to be asked of a woman in labor to gain information to help assess the situation including due date, if there are any known issues with the pregnancy (such as breech position), or participation in prenatal care. Information regarding timing of contractions and degree of pain should also be obtained. The presence of bleeding or any type of discharge is important to note. The mother should be questioned about the type of pressure she is feeling in her abdominal area as well as if she is feeling the urge to start pushing. All of this information coupled with whether the baby's head is crowning will help in determining transport viability.

10. D: In treating an ankle or foot injury, stabilize the limb, taking care not to change the position of the ankle, and tie a pillow to the ankle and foot. Do not apply manual traction or put an ice pack directly on the skin.

11. C: You form a general impression during the first few seconds of contact with the patient. The most important determination is the presence of any life-threatening condition or injury. If the patient is injured or ill, "sick" or "not sick," is initially determined by observing and you can prioritize and form a plan of action. At this point, you do not have adequate information to determine a diagnosis or transport the patient.

12. A: If trauma is suspected on an unconscious patient, care must be taken to prevent spinal damage. The jaw thrust technique (also known as anterior mandible displacement technique) is the best choice for manually opening the airway. When a patient is unconscious, muscle control of the jaw is suspended, making the jaw easy to open. The index fingers are positioned behind the angle of the jaw, and the jaw is then pushed upward. The tips of the thumbs can be used to keep the jaw in an open position. This allows the head to remain in a neutral position instead of flexed or extended, where damage to the spine could potentially occur.

13. B: Expressed consent is providing direct confirmation by the patient that treatment can be provided. The patient must be of legal age in order to provide consent. In many states, this is the age that one is considered an adult and is usually around the age of 18. There may be several exceptions to this rule, including a minor who is pregnant, married, or legally emancipated. The person must also be able to make a decision that considers the implications or consequences of proposed treatment. If the patient is mentally incapacitated for any reason, such as dementia or drug or alcohol ingestion, then expressed consent cannot be given. In cases such as this, implied consent may be assumed or may be given by a spouse or other close family member. The other criteria would be that the patient or legal guardian understands the risks and benefits of the proposed treatment. Treatment cannot commence until the criteria have been met.

14. A: Vaginal bleeding that occurs late in pregnancy is usually related to an issue with the placenta. If bleeding is accompanied by severe abdominal pain in the lower abdominal region, it may be due to placental abruption, in which the placenta separates from the uterine wall. Any amount of placental separation from the uterine wall occurs in about 1 out of 150 live births. Placenta previa can also be a possibility where the placenta is positioned low in the uterus and may sometimes cover the cervical opening. As the cervix begins to thin as pregnancy progresses, it may cause bleeding. Any bleeding late in pregnancy can be dangerous. The patient should be treated for the symptoms she is showing. Because of the bleeding and potential for complications, advanced life support (ALS) should be called to assist. Oxygen should be administered through a nonrebreather mask, she should be positioned on her left side to relieve pressure on the vena cava, and the patient should be observed for signs of shock.

15. A: Angina is the medical term that describes chest pain that follows exertion and results from poor oxygenation of the cardiac muscle. Dyspnea refers to difficulty in breathing. Congestive heart failure is the term used for a form of heart failure in which the heart is unable to pump out the returning blood quickly enough, resulting in congestion in the veins and fluid build-up in the lungs. Tachycardia is the medical term for a fast heart rate.

16. D: Fibrillation is the condition in which the heart muscle fibers are producing uncontrolled rapid contractions. During fibrillation, the heart cannot produce a pulse. Ventricular tachycardia refers to a heart rate of more than 100 beats per minute in which the beat originates in the ventricles. Atrial tachycardia is a condition in which the beat originates in the atrium and the rate per minute is above the normal range. Heart block is a condition in which the nerve impulses that control the heartbeat are irregular, and this causes the atria and ventricles to stop beating in the same rhythm.

17. B: If any pulse is palpable, do not use the AED. It is appropriate to use when the patient is unresponsive and there is no detectable pulse or respiration.

18. C: Normally, amniotic fluid is clear; a greenish or brownish color may indicate maternal or fetal distress. Bleeding does not accompany breakage of the amniotic sac.

19. B: Obstruction of the airway is a dangerous situation. The obstruction can be complete or partial. If the airway is completely blocked, the child will not be able to speak and will become cyanotic (blue). In a child, back blows are not performed. Back blows can be performed on an infant if the infant is held in the facedown position while supporting the head and neck. In an older child, a finger sweep can be done if the foreign object is seen in the airway. If no foreign objects are seen, abdominal thrusts can be performed. If the child is unresponsive, it is important to try to ventilate the child as you are trying to locate the foreign object.

20. D: When you make an error on a report, strike through the mistake with a single horizontal line, initial beside the strikeout, and then write the correct information. Never erase, use correction fluid, or obliterate with multiple lines any information on a medical report.

21. A: When releasing chest compression, the chest wall must fully recoil to allow the heart to fill completely. For maximum effectiveness, you should maintain straight arms with locked elbows, and lift at the hips while maintaining light contact on the patient. Bending the elbows does not allow for maximal strength in chest compressions. Full contact does not need to be removed and will add time between compressions. This may also result in administering compressions in the incorrect and/or inconsistent location on the chest.

22. C: If the patient has a pulse, but has stopped breathing, rescue breaths should be administered. Chest compressions are not required if the patient has a pulse. If the patient has stopped breathing and has no pulse, initiate CPR. Blind sweeps are not recommended in respiratory arrest, as they risk pushing something further into the airway.

23. D: When the description of the patient includes "AOx3," or "Alert and Oriented times three," this is a reference to the patient's correct response to who he is, where he is, and what day it is. It does not refer to the patient's ability to ambulate.

24. B: There are three layers of skin: epidermis, dermis, and subcutaneous or hypodermis. The epidermis is the outermost layer of skin. The dermis continually regenerates and serves as an overall protective barrier to the body. Injuries to this layer are usually superficial and heal quickly. The epidermal layer will gradually begin to thin during the aging process. The dermis is the middle layer. The dermis contains the blood vessels, nerve endings, sweat glands, and oil-secreting glands. If a skin injury occurs in this layer, pain will result. The third layer is the subcutaneous layer, where fat deposition occurs. An injury to this layer will have even more pain and bleeding.

25. D: Any patient who may potentially have an injury to the neck or cervical spine needs to be immobilized before transport in order to prevent additional injuries. A cervical collar or cervical spinal immobilization device is placed around the neck. It is typically used in conjunction with a long or short backboard. The correct size collar should be used so it fits the patient appropriately. The base of the collar should be on the patient's chest, and the chin should fit comfortably on the chin rest and should not be able to move. A long spine board or backboard is used to immobilize from the head all the way to the pelvic area and extremities. It is used with patients who are lying down. The short backboard is used for patients who are sitting down. There are several types that include vest-like boards and rigid short boards. Sometimes the long and short boards are used together. Proper use of these devices is essential to prevent further injury.

26. B: Even with proper placement and confirmation, an endotracheal tube can easily become dislodged. Any time the patient is moved, such as during loading or unloading from the ambulance, the patient himself moves his body or head, or the tube is not secured, it is possible for the tube to become dislodged. This can be very dangerous for the patient, because it prevents proper ventilation from occurring and puts the patient at risk for the complications of oxygen deprivation. The paramedic should be alerted to assess tube placement. The tube can be secured using tape, and the patient can also be placed in a cervical collar to help with controlling head movements. Vital signs should be checked after each time the patient is moved.

27. C: Defibrillation makes the greatest difference in survival of the cardiac arrest patient. IV therapy and oxygen administration are important, but the most important action is defibrillation. Nitroglycerin is a drug used for relief of angina.

28. B: When describing the area of an extremity that is near the trunk, the correct term is proximal. Distal refers to an area away, or distant, from the trunk. Posterior means toward the back, and lateral means away from the midline.

29. A: This patient has the appearance of classic emphysema. Emphysema is a type of chronic obstructive pulmonary disease (COPD) caused by smoking or chronic exposure to cigarette smoke or other noxious fumes. This disease works to destroy the surface of the alveoli, making it difficult for gas exchange to occur. As a result, the patient must adapt compensatory breathing strategies in order to get enough oxygen. The shape of the patient's chest will change over time to look like a barrel. The patient will also breathe through pursed lips and will appear to be puffing instead of taking normal breaths. Because breathing is difficult, more calories are burned during the process, and these patients tend to have difficulty maintaining or gaining weight. As this disease advances, any type of exertion will be difficult. Inhalers and chronic oxygen use are common. It is important to look for signs of active cigarette smoking while using oxygen, as this is an extremely dangerous situation.

30. A: Activated charcoal acts by binding to certain poisons and keeping them from being absorbed in the stomach.

31. A: Respiratory distress is a condition that will be frequently seen as an EMT. The very first step that should be taken when treating a patient with breathing difficulty is to administer oxygen. This is typically administered via a nonrebreather mask at 15 liters/minute. After the patient is receiving oxygen, the focused history and physical examination can begin. The questions in the focused history will follow the acronym OPQRST (onset, provocation, quality of the distress, radiation of pain, severity of distress, time the respiratory distress started). The physical exam will involve taking and recording vital signs. The most important step, however, is the initiation of oxygen therapy because individuals of any age cannot be without oxygen for very long without suffering from irreversible damage.

32. D: Baseline vital signs are extremely important when first assessing a patient. The first step in monitoring the patient is to observe trends in vital signs. The respiratory rate is a measure of how fast or slow an individual is breathing. The normal range for an adult is 12 to 20 breaths per minute and will vary for children, but a newborn typically breathes faster at 40 to 60 breaths per minute (bpm); a 3-year-old, 25 to 30 bpm; a 5- to 7-year-old, 20 to 25 bpm; and a 10- to 15-year-old, 15 to 20. The pulse rate is the number of heartbeats in one minute. A normal pulse rate also varies, but for a newborn it is 120 to 160; 3-year-old, 80 to 120; 5- to 10-year-old, 70 to 115; 15-year-old, 70 to 90; and an adult is 60 to 80. Blood pressure is a measure of the force on the arteries in the heart as it relaxes and contracts, and the reading will vary. The 16-year-old in the question has an elevated pulse and respiratory rate and a low blood pressure.

33. C: All industrial facilities must keep Safety Data Sheets (SDSs) that describe the chemicals they use and the first-aid treatments for exposure to those chemicals.

34. B: Never administer oral glucose to an unconscious patient who cannot protect their airway.

35. B: The normal pulse rate for an adult is between 60 and 100 beats per minute. In an emergency situation, the pulse rate may rise to between 100 and 140 beats per minute. A pulse rate below 50 beats per minute indicates a serious problem.

36. B: Osteoporosis is the most common bone disease, and it is estimated that at least half of women over the age of 50 have this condition. Approximately 20% of men will also have this condition. Osteoporosis is caused by gradual thinning of the bone and loss of bone density. It can be due to a number of reasons including age; lack of calcium, phosphorus, and vitamin D in the diet; genetic predisposition; low body weight; smoking; alcohol use; and lack of physical activity. Postmenopausal women are also at higher risk due to a reduction in estrogen levels. Any individual with osteoporosis is at risk for fractures. In the elderly, even a short fall can cause a fracture.

37. B: A hip fracture is a fracture of the proximal femur, not the pelvis.

38. A: Many patients have designated themselves as organ donors upon death. This is often indicated on the patient's driver's license or may be indicated on a donor card. A legal document must be available and signed by the organ donor specifying wishes for organ donation. As an EMT, medical care must continue to be provided at the appropriate level, regardless of whether the patient is an organ donor. A wish to donate organs upon death is important, but the wish cannot be honored until death occurs. Unless the patient has a DNR order on record, all life-sustaining treatment should be offered and attempted. If this does not happen, the EMT could potentially be held responsible for negligence. The main concern is always saving the patient's life. The organ donation designation comes second.

39. D: Consuming even small amounts of iron can be life-threatening in children. Usual signs of iron poisoning include nausea, diarrhea, and bloody vomiting.

40. B: Your first step is to protect the patient from staring bystanders, asking them to leave in a polite but firm manner. Next, you should help the patient to remove any clothing that obstructs your view of the vaginal opening. A feeling of an impending bowel movement and bulging at the vaginal opening indicate that birth is imminent; however, the patient should not be allowed to use the bathroom. Because the baby may be born any minute, transport is not practical at this time.

41. C: Visible bulging at the vaginal opening indicates that crowning is taking place and that birth is imminent. At this point, it is not practical to transport the patient. Instead, you should gently position the mother in the cab with one foot resting on the seat and the other on the floor and prepare for delivery.

42. A: The baby should be supported throughout the entire birth process. Place one hand below the baby's head as it delivers. Tell the mother not to push while you check to make sure the umbilical cord is not wrapped around the baby's neck. Never pull on the baby during delivery. Grasping a slippery baby by the feet may cause you to drop the child.

43. B: Hemorrhagic shock is the medical term for hypoperfusion due to a massive hemorrhage (loss of blood). Hypovolemic shock differs from hemorrhagic shock in that the volume in the circulatory system is low due to the loss of bodily fluid from dehydration, diarrhea, vomiting, or significant burns. Cardiogenic shock refers to hypoperfusion due to a cardiac cause.

44. A: Always make sure the patient has been decontaminated before transporting him or her to the hospital; a contaminated patient or EMT can contaminate the entire ambulance team. If a patient requires immediate life-saving care, even if he or she has not been decontaminated, you should provide that care, being careful to wear protective clothing and to decontaminate yourself as soon as possible.

45. A: Never attempt to suck the venom from a snakebite. Do not put ice on the bite unless instructed to do so by a physician or local protocol. The bite should be cleaned with soap and water and the patient transported to the hospital immediately.

46. C: A tracheostomy is a surgical opening in the neck and into the trachea to allow for breathing. A tracheotomy is the surgical procedure to create this opening. A tracheostomy is needed for certain patients to help with breathing with a ventilator over the long term. Many pediatric patients have tracheotomies and live at home with the parents providing care for them. The parents become well versed in taking care of the tracheostomy tube, but occasionally the tube becomes dislodged and needs to be reinserted at the hospital. If the child is unable to breathe in the interim, the EMT may need to help ventilate the patient until admission to the hospital. The first choice is to cover the stoma or opening in the neck. The bag-valve-mask should be placed over the mouth and nose, and the patient can be ventilated. If this is not possible, the second choice would be to ventilate using a smaller mask over the stoma while keeping the patient's mouth closed.

47. C: The preeminent sign of hypoperfusion is the change in mental status.

48. A: First, you should assume your position above the patient's head. If a second EMT is available to assist you, he or she should stabilize the head and neck. When working alone, use your knees to keep the head from moving. Use a mask, and preserve the seal by placing the thumb and index fingers on top of the mask, with the middle, ring, and little fingers placed firmly under the chin.

Once the mask is in place, use the jaw thrust to open the airway. Do not apply pressure to the chin, because this may occlude the airway.

49. C: Because the patient has been lying in the cold all night, he is most likely suffering from hypothermia. Signs of hypothermia include muscular rigidity, amnesia, and loss of contact with environment.

50. D: The best course of action to prevent additional body heat loss in an injured patient trapped in a cold environment is to create a barrier to the cold. Blankets or articles of clothing can be used to protect the patient from exposure to wind or water. Active rewarming may result in cardiac arrest, and ingestion of stimulants may result in impaired circulation.

51. A: Individuals under the influence of alcohol or drugs may be more susceptible to hypothermia. The fact that the patient had been drinking and was trapped overnight in a cold environment places him at high risk of hypothermia.

52. C: Negligence is an injury that occurs as a direct result of an error or omission by an EMT that is a normal standard of care or practice. The key is deciding what would usually be done in a certain situation by an EMT with similar training and experience. In order for negligence to have occurred, four criteria must be present. The first is duty to act. The EMT must have failed to provide emergency services. The second is breach of duty. The EMT must have failed to provide the appropriate level of service that another EMT would have provided in the same type of case and with similar training, education, and experience. The third is that the patient incurred some type of injury. The last criterion is that the patient incurred this injury as a direct result of the EMT's action or omission. All four of these must be met in order for negligence to be considered.

53. A: The correct range for the pulse of a five-year-old is 70 to 115.

54. D: In removing an injured child from a car safety seat, apply a cervical collar to maintain manual stabilization of the head and neck. Do not slide the child out of the seat or strap the child to the backboard across the abdomen. Taping the child across the chin may put pressure on the neck.

55. B: A patient may have a DNR order on file with their primary care physician and the local hospital. Many times, an EMT responding to a call will not have immediate access to this information. If written documentation cannot be produced at the time of cardiac or respiratory arrest, CPR must be initiated. Patients may submit copies of a DNR order to the local EMS in order to help with decision making. Another point to note is that if the patient or the durable power of attorney has second thoughts about life-sustaining treatment at the time treatment is needed, treatment cannot be withheld. It is important to learn the exact local or state guidelines or regulations about providing life-sustaining treatment and the EMS role. These regulations regarding these advanced directives will vary from state to state or county to county.

56. B: Precautions need to always be taken to protect oneself from direct contact with any bodily substances such as blood or waste products. These precautions include mask, gown, eye protection, and gloves. The next step would be to immediately assess the airway in order to ventilate the patient with high-flow oxygen. This helps to minimize damage to the body due to oxygen deprivation. Standard procedure should be followed in assessing and establishing the airway. The patient may also require suctioning to clear any material, such as blood, from the airway. The next step should then be to try to stop or control the bleeding to prevent further blood loss. If there are no lower body injuries, the legs may be elevated 8 to 12 inches to try to increase blood flow to the brain. If lower body injuries are present, the patient should be maintained in a neutral position. The patient should also be prevented from losing body heat by covering him or her with a blanket.

57. D: A contusion, or bruise, is a closed injury of the soft tissue in which there is cellular damage and discoloration of the dermis. Laceration and abrasion are both open injuries. Concussion is a closed injury involving the brain.

58. C: One of the most challenging skills to learn is proper placement of an endotracheal tube, and it is one of the most important. If an endotracheal tube is properly inserted, you should be able to hear breath sounds in the lungs and over the epigastric region. If gurgling sounds are heard, this is an indication that the tube is in the esophagus and needs to be immediately corrected, or the patient can die. The cuff should be deflated, the endotracheal tube should be removed, and the patient should be ventilated to prevent hypoxia. If breath sounds are only audible on one side of the lungs, the tube may be too far down and is likely to be located in the right main stem bronchi. Other ways to check placement include pulse oximetry to monitor oxygen saturation levels.

59. D: When a patient has a spinal cord injury, the blood vessels below the injury site stop constricting and dilate due to neurogenic shock. Anaphylactic shock is the result of a severe allergic reaction. Septic shock occurs in the presence of an overwhelming infection. Hypovolemic shock is hypoperfusion due to fluid volume loss from diarrhea, dehydration, vomiting, or significant burns.

60. D: Never rub or squeeze a frostbitten or frozen area, as this can seriously damage the injured tissue. Active rewarming is seldom recommended in cases of frostbite or freezing because of the risk of permanent injury. You should administer high-concentration oxygen, cover the frozen or frostbitten area, and transport the patient to the hospital immediately.

61. B: If transport is delayed and the local protocol recommends it, begin active rewarming of the frozen area, taking care that the injured area does not touch the sides or bottom of the container. Never massage or rub snow on a frostbitten or frozen area. Patients should not be allowed to smoke or drink alcoholic beverages because of the risk of decreasing circulation.

62. C: Active external rewarming is the process of applying heat externally in the treatment of mild to moderate hypothermia (a core temperature of 30–37.1 °C or 86–98.7 °F) and recent studies have even shown effectiveness in the context of severe hypothermia. This method includes using warm blankets, forced air, warm IV fluids, and applying warmed water bottles to the axilla and groin where large vessels are closest to the body's surface. Studies have shown the risk for "afterdrop" after active external rewarming, or a return to suboptimal body temperature after the warming method is discontinued due to cold blood in the extremities moving through circulation. Active internal rewarming measures are reserved for severe hypothermia with cardiac arrest and include invasive measures such as warming the blood through dialysis or ECMO.

63. B: The preferred method for moving a patient down stairs is to use a stair chair or wheeled stretcher. This method is usually safer and more efficient than the others mentioned.

64. B: Mouth-to-mask ventilation is the method that is preferred over other types of ventilation in the field. This is a relatively simple method to perform. The benefit is that both hands are free to make a tight seal around the mouth, enabling the best ventilator volume possible. Mouth-to-mouth ventilation is not a preferred method because of the direct contact with the patient and the inability to protect oneself adequately from body substances. The two-person bag-valve-mask utilizes a self-inflating bag along with a mask. Two EMTs are required to perform this type of ventilation, and the benefit is that 90% to 100% oxygen can be administered when hooked up to an oxygen source. A one-person valve mask is more difficult to use because one person is required to keep the mask sealed while compressing the bag to deliver oxygen.

65. A: One of the reasons that it is important to maintain body temperature during shock is to help preserve oxygen and energy. As the body temperature drops, the body will begin to shiver, which will use valuable oxygen and energy in the process. This oxygen could be better used for preventing organ and brain damage. This needs to occur even in warm or hot temperatures. Low body temperature is a sign of shock as well as cold, clammy skin. The cool and clammy skin is due the action of epinephrine and norepinephrine, which are secreted by the adrenal gland in response to the stress of losing blood. This causes vasoconstriction to occur.

66. D: Signs or symptoms indicative of an acute psychological problem following a stressful event include uncontrollable crying, inappropriate behavior, or irrational thoughts; however, nausea, loss of appetite, or difficulty sleeping are typical reactions and usually do not require intervention.

67. D: Stabbing pain in the chest that increases in intensity with deep breaths is usually associated with the respiratory system. Cardiac pain is characteristically a crushing or pressure type of discomfort. GI upset and gallbladder disease may cause pain in the center of the chest or back or under the right rib cage.

68. D: Manufacturer's instructions should be verified on strap use, but EMTs are taught the following basic procedure. Straps are color coded on the KED for simplifying use. There are two head straps, two leg straps, and three chest straps. First, the chest straps are applied in the order of middle and bottom. The thigh or leg straps are secured next. The head is secured, followed by tightening of the top strap. Ensure that the patient is able to breathe properly and that the strap is not too tight. There are a couple of mnemonics that are used: "My Baby Looks Hot Tonight" or "Money Buys Lots of Hot Toys," in which the first letter of each word helps you to remember the order. The main point to remember is that the head should be secured after the middle to prevent additional injuries from occurring.

69. C: Tachypnea is the medical term used for shallow, fast breathing. A normal respiratory rate is somewhere around 12 to 20 breaths per minute for an adult. Breathing faster than 24 breaths per minute is considered tachypnea. Tachypnea can be caused by many different illnesses, including pneumonia, asthma, chronic obstructive pulmonary disease (COPD), chest pain, or pulmonary embolism. Patients who are breathing rapidly should be administered oxygen at a rate of 15 liters/minute. A nonrebreather mask can be used, or in some cases, a nasal cannula may be substituted. Patients who have a history of asthma or COPD may need to use their inhaler as well to help open up the airway.

70. D: It is imperative to use a *water-soluble lubricant* when inserting any type of airway, because a petroleum-based lubricant could enter the lung and cause lipid pneumonia. The correct method for measuring a nasopharyngeal airway is to measure the distance between the tip of the nose and the earlobe. Position the bevel of the airway toward the base of the nose or the septum.

71. B: In some states, an off-duty EMT has no legal obligation to provide care; however, you may feel a moral obligation to help a patient in need. It is always best to provide care and contact other emergency personnel for additional help. Leaving the scene of an accident, even after providing care, may be construed as abandoning a patient.

72. B: The first step in treating a patient with potential cardiac arrest is to administer oxygen. At that point, you should obtain a patient history and perform a physical exam to obtain baseline vital signs.

73. D: When a patient loses consciousness, the first step is to open the airway. If you find the patient to be in cardiac arrest based on your initial assessment, you should attach an automated external defibrillator.

74. B: In addition to administering oxygen, the most effective way to decrease oxygen demand is to calm and reassure the patient. Driving at high speeds, flashing lights, or turning on the siren will only heighten the patient's distress.

75. D: The blow-by oxygen technique is an alternative for administering oxygen to a child who is afraid of having a mask on their face. Nasal and oral airways or endotracheal tubes are applicable only if the child is unresponsive.

76. D: When assessing the newborn's heart rate, if it is less than 100 beats per minute, the bradycardia algorithm should be followed. With a heart beat of less than 100, but greater than 60, the newborn should be monitored, given oxygen, and a 12-lead EKG obtained. If the heart rate drops under 60 beats per minute, chest compressions should be given. There are special standards for conducting CPR on a newborn, and these guidelines should be followed. Once the heart rate is above 60, free-flow oxygen should be administered by holding the oxygen mask close to the baby's mouth but not placing it directly on the face.

77. A: Altered mental status is the condition in which a patient responds inappropriately, either verbally or nonverbally. A seizure is a sudden attack caused by a random discharge of electrical current in the brain; it usually results in a temporary altered mental status. A coma is a prolonged episode of deep unconsciousness. Hypoglycemia is a serious and sudden drop in blood sugar levels in which the patient may appear to be intoxicated, shaky, diaphoretic, and clammy.

78. A: The stage of labor in which the head of the baby is showing in the vaginal orifice is crowning. Pushing is the term used for the act of bearing down as if having a bowel movement. Bloody show refers to the expulsion of the mucous plug because of cervical dilation in the beginning of labor. Dilation is the act of opening of the cervix during labor to allow for expulsion of the baby.

EMT Practice Test #2

1. Which of the following statements regarding consent is FALSE?

    a. Care may be given to a child without parental consent.
    b. Expressed consent must be given by all patients before treatment is given.
    c. In the case of an unconscious patient, consent may be assumed.
    d. A mentally impaired patient has the right to refuse treatment.

2. Your teenage patient has a nosebleed and appears extremely distraught. Which of the following treatment methods is inappropriate?

    a. Lean the patient forward.
    b. Pinch the fleshy skin at the lower portion of the nose.
    c. Place the patient in the Trendelenburg position (lying back with feet up).
    d. Keep the patient calm and quiet.

3. When assessing a patient with a possible spinal injury, which of the following is something you should NEVER do?

    a. Ask the patient if they feel any areas of tenderness.
    b. If the patient is not in pain, ask them to move their back to see what the response is.
    c. Position yourself in front of the patient while asking them questions.
    d. Ask the patient to grab your hands and squeeze.

4. As you prepare to place an endotracheal tube, all of the following are important steps to take before placing the endotracheal tube EXCEPT:

    a. Put on gloves, mask, and eye protection to protect yourself from potentially hazardous bodily fluids.
    b. Check the cuff for possible leaks by inflating the balloon and squeezing gently to make sure air is not escaping.
    c. Insert the stylus into the tube.
    d. Select the proper tube diameter, which in most cases is an 8.5 to 9 mm diameter.

5. Which category does a patient with a blood glucose level of 70 or below fall within?

    a. Hyperglycemic
    b. Normal range
    c. Hypoglycemic
    d. Diabetic

Refer to the following for questions 6-8:

> You receive a call from a distraught 18-year-old girl. Her parents are away for the weekend and she is having an illicit party during which alcohol and other substances have been consumed. Her 16-year-old brother has slipped and hit his head on the coffee table. The boy has a contusion on the side of his head. He is conscious but has slurred speech and appears confused. He denies having consumed any alcohol or drugs.

6. In addition to alcohol intoxication, what might slurred speech and confusion be signs of?

    a. Altered mental state
    b. Head injury
    c. Seizure
    d. Drug overdose

7. What is the best course of action in this case?

    a. Transport the patient to the hospital.
    b. Call the police.
    c. Ask the patient again if he has been using drugs.
    d. Call the parents.

8. The patient suddenly becomes violent and begins to throw objects around the room. What should your reaction be?

    a. Reassure the patient.
    b. Restrain the patient.
    c. Go to a safe place and call the police.
    d. Call the parents.

9. Which of the following statements regarding use of visual warning devices in an emergency vehicle is FALSE?

    a. Headlights should be kept on both day and night.
    b. Four-way flashers can be used as emergency lights.
    c. Alternating flashing headlights should only be used if attached to secondary head lamps.
    d. Lights should blink in tandem rather than in an alternating pattern.

10. Which of the following describes a scrape in which the top layers of the skin are missing?

    a. Contusion
    b. Puncture
    c. Laceration
    d. Abrasion

11. Which of the following statements regarding burns is FALSE?

    a. Chemical burns can burn continuously for days.
    b. Alkaline chemicals can enter the bloodstream via burns.
    c. The age of the patient should be considered when assessing burns.
    d. An electrical burn is usually not serious.

12. You are assessing a pregnant patient who appears to be close to term. She is having regular contractions, and upon examination, you decide she is in the second stage of labor. What would be the BEST indication of this?

    a. Regular contractions 10 minutes apart
    b. Evidence of bloody show
    c. Crowning is evident
    d. The cervix is dilated almost to 10 cm

13. Which of the following is the most frequently seen symptom of acute respiratory distress?

   a. Cyanosis
   b. Absent breath sounds
   c. Rapid or slow respiratory rate
   d. Change in level of consciousness

14. All of the following are symptoms of hypoglycemia EXCEPT:

   a. Hunger
   b. Sweating
   c. Frequent urination
   d. Confusion or disorientation

15. What is the acronym to use when performing a trauma assessment?

   a. DCAP-LETS
   b. CAP-BLT
   c. DCAP-BTLS
   d. BDIP-BTLS

Refer to the following for questions 16-18:

> The mother of a 4-year-old boy calls you because her son is running a high fever. The boy has been vomiting and has diarrhea. His temperature is 103 °F.

16. What is the best line of treatment for a child with diarrhea and vomiting?

   a. Allow the child to sip some water or chipped ice.
   b. Maintain an open airway and administer oxygen.
   c. Insert an oropharyngeal airway.
   d. Administer an antidiarrheal.

17. What is the first step in assessing a child with fever?

   a. Obtain an oral temperature.
   b. Obtain a rectal temperature.
   c. Determine the child's temperature using a skin thermometer.
   d. Cover the child with towels soaked in tepid water.

18. On transport to the hospital, the child suddenly has a seizure. What should you do immediately?

   a. Provide oxygen.
   b. Insert an oropharyngeal airway.
   c. Insert a bite stick.
   d. Keep the child covered and wait until arrival at the hospital.

19. In which patients may activated charcoal be safely used?

   a. Patients with altered mental status
   b. Patients who have ingested acid
   c. Patients who have ingested gasoline
   d. Patients who have ingested aspirin

20. Which of the following statements regarding a twin birth is FALSE?

a. There may be a separate placenta for each baby.
b. The second baby may deliver in a breech position.
c. The placenta delivers only after the second twin is born.
d. The umbilical cord of the first twin should be cut before the second twin is born.

21. What is the best way to save an avulsed body part?

a. Put the part in dry ice.
b. Immerse the part in ice water.
c. Wrap the part in a dry sterile dressing.
d. Immerse the part in saline.

22. What should you do to treat an open abdominal injury?

a. Apply an occlusive dressing using aluminum foil.
b. Replace any eviscerated or exposed organs.
c. Give the patient sips of water.
d. Apply a sterile saline dressing.

23. A 22-year-old man was riding his bicycle. He hit a bump and fell off his bike into the street. A passing car ran over his leg. What kind of leg injury did he likely sustain from the car?

a. Laceration
b. Contusion
c. Avulsion
d. Closed crush injury

24. Which of the following would be a violation of confidentiality?

a. Providing information to a police officer for a suspected rape situation
b. Giving a medical update to a neighbor who is on the scene while treatment is occurring
c. Calling authorities to report that a patient has been bitten by a potentially rabid raccoon
d. Providing information to the nurse admitting the patient in the emergency room

25. You arrive at a large swimming pool where a 14-year-old boy is floating in the water supported by several people. The lifeguard informs you that the boy hit his head on the diving board as he attempted a dive, and he was unable to move after he entered the water. Which action is inappropriate?

a. Place the boy on a long backboard while he is still in the water.
b. Apply a cervical spine immobilization device.
c. Have the people who are supporting the boy lift him out of the water.
d. Strap the boy onto the long backboard with two or more straps.

26. Which term refers to a serious allergic reaction that could be life threatening?

a. Anaphylaxis
b. Ronchi
c. Edema
d. Epistaxis

27. You arrive at the scene of a car vs. pedestrian accident and observe that the victim has a major laceration of the thigh with extensive bleeding. He is lying on the ground and appears unresponsive. What is your first action?

 a. Don protective gloves, and apply direct pressure on the wound.
 b. Don protective gloves, and assess the airway and breathing.
 c. Don protective gloves, and start CPR.
 d. Don protective gloves, and apply an upper thigh tourniquet.

28. Which of the following drugs can an EMT assist a patient in taking?

 a. Nitroglycerin
 b. Amitriptyline
 c. Verapamil
 d. Nifedipine

29. You respond to a call for a three-year-old boy who pulled a pot of boiling soup off the stove. When you assess the child, you observe blistering over his entire face, neck, and trunk of the body. What is your main goal?

 a. Ensure a patent airway and transport immediately.
 b. Apply sterile saline or water, sterile dressings, and then transport.
 c. Apply antibiotic ointment, dry dressing, and then transport.
 d. Wrap the patient in warm blankets and transport.

30. How does a child's airway differ from an adult's?

 a. The tongue is smaller.
 b. The chest wall is more rigid.
 c. The tongue is larger.
 d. The trachea is wider.

31. What do the signs and symptoms of carbon monoxide poisoning most closely resemble?

 a. Smoke inhalation
 b. Flu
 c. Food poisoning
 d. Drug overdose

32. How should you open the airway of an unconscious patient with a possible spinal injury?

 a. Perform the head-tilt maneuver.
 b. Perform the chin-lift maneuver.
 c. Rotate the patient's head.
 d. Perform the jaw-thrust maneuver.

33. In the case of a patient with chronic bronchitis in respiratory distress, what is the preferred course of action?

 a. Withhold oxygen.
 b. Provide artificial ventilation.
 c. Place the patient in a supine position.
 d. Administer oxygen.

34. Typical changes to a woman's body during late pregnancy include which of the following?
    a. Increased blood pressure
    b. Increased cardiac output
    c. Reduced heart rate
    d. Reduced blood volume

35. In which of the following patients is rapid trauma assessment most urgently needed?
    a. A 90-year-old woman with pain in the right upper quadrant
    b. A conscious 50-year-old man who fell from the roof of his home and landed on his left arm
    c. A conscious 25-year-old store clerk who was stabbed in the abdomen during an attempted robbery
    d. An 8-year-old boy complaining of pain in the right lower quadrant of the abdomen

36. Which of the following is likely to be the sublingual dosage for nitroglycerin?
    a. 0.3 mg
    b. 0.1 mg
    c. 3 mg
    d. 1 g

37. In rescuing a near-drowning victim, what should you do?
    a. Perform chest compression.
    b. Attempt rescue breathing while the victim is still in the water.
    c. Remove the victim from the water before initiating care.
    d. Immobilize the victim, then remove the victim from the water.

38. You arrive at the home of a snakebite patient. Which of the following actions is inappropriate?
    a. Administer oxygen.
    b. Have suction available.
    c. Immobilize the affected extremity.
    d. Catch the snake for identification.

Refer to the following for questions 39-41:

> You receive a call from the mother of a 3-year-old girl. The mother believes her daughter has "swallowed something." When you arrive, the child does not acknowledge your presence. She has a high fever and a generalized rash.

39. What does proper care for a small child with possible airway obstruction consist of?
    a. Performing a finger sweep
    b. Relieving mild airway obstruction
    c. Avoiding agitation of the child and providing transport
    d. Applying back blows and abdominal thrusts

40. When a young child does not acknowledge the presence of a stranger in his or her environment, what is this indicative of?
    a. Altered mental state
    b. Allergic reaction
    c. Sleep
    d. Age-appropriate behavior

41. What should a child with inattentive behavior, high fever, and generalized rash be monitored for?

    a. Dehydration
    b. Projectile vomiting
    c. Cardiac failure
    d. Seizures

42. When you assess a patient's blood loss, which of the following is inaccurate?

    a. The smaller the patient, the less blood volume is present.
    b. The smaller the patient, the lower the amount of bleeding that will cause shock.
    c. A child loses blood at a slower rate than an adult does.
    d. A young adult tolerates blood loss better than an older adult does.

43. You arrive at the home of a young couple who have an unresponsive one-month-old baby. Upon examination, you see that the baby is in rigor mortis (the rigid stiffening of the muscles after death). What is your next action?

    a. CPR
    b. Intubate the baby, and then transport
    c. Comfort the parents
    d. Use the defibrillator, and then start CPR

44. Types of bronchodilators include all of the following EXCEPT:

    a. Alupent
    b. Pulmicort
    c. Proventil
    d. Metaprel

45. Which of the following conditions often presents with emesis that contains black particles that appear like "coffee grounds"?

    a. Bleeding from the colon
    b. Bleeding from the bladder
    c. Bleeding from the respiratory system
    d. Bleeding from the stomach

46. What is the approximate FiO_2 of a patient receiving 5 Lpm of oxygen by nasal cannula?

    a. 32%
    b. 40%
    c. 44%
    d. 50%

47. A full oxygen tank is pressurized at about 2,000 pounds per square inch. Which technique for transporting oxygen is appropriate?

    a. Secure tanks to prevent falling and rolling during transport.
    b. Wrap tanks with blankets to prevent contact with other tanks.
    c. Lift tanks by their valves and gauges.
    d. Oxygen tanks are not inherently dangerous, so no special precautions are necessary.

48. You respond to a call where a six-year-old boy is experiencing an allergic reaction to a bee sting. Upon arrival, you observe that the child is loudly wheezing and appears to have facial edema. The mother informs you that he has an epinephrine autoinjector pen because of a peanut allergy. What is the appropriate action?

   a. Administer the epinephrine.
   b. Call for medical direction.
   c. Transport the patient without giving the epinephrine.
   d. Have the child administer the epinephrine.

49. Emergency care for a burn patient includes which of the following treatments?

   a. Apply cold sterile saline or sterile water to the burn.
   b. Cover the burn with a clean, dry dressing
   c. Apply ointment to the burn to soothe and prevent scarring.
   d. Keep the patient cool during transport to prevent additional burn damage.

50. You are attempting to ventilate a nonbreathing patient who has a tracheal stoma. If ventilation through the stoma results in air escaping through the mouth and nose, what is your next action?

   a. Suction the stoma.
   b. Close the mouth and pinch the nose.
   c. Cover the stoma and ventilate through the mouth.
   d. Insert a nasopharyngeal airway.

51. What does proper care of an injury to the fibula or tibia include?

   a. Treating for shock
   b. Applying an ice pack
   c. Applying wet heat
   d. Applying manual traction

52. Which of the following is NOT a true statement?

   a. The oropharyngeal airway should be selected for an unconscious patient.
   b. The oropharyngeal airway is a better choice for a patient who is having seizures.
   c. A conscious patient is likely to experience the gag reflex with the use of an oropharyngeal airway.
   d. The nasopharyngeal airway is less likely to stimulate the gag reflex.

53. On each side of the face there is a structure composed of a slender bar of bone that connects the temporal bone to the cheekbone. What is the medical term for this formation?

   a. Mandible
   b. Maxilla
   c. Orbit
   d. Zygomatic arch

Refer to the following for questions 54-56:

> The sister of an 80-year-old man reports that her brother is bleeding profusely. On arrival, the man is conscious and lying on the couch with his legs up. The seat of his pants is soaked in blood, as are the towels placed underneath. The patient states

that he is bleeding from his rectum. The bleeding began after dinner, when he felt a sharp pain in his lower abdomen.

54. What is severe blood loss in an adult defined as?

    a. 150 cc
    b. 250 cc
    c. 500 cc
    d. 1,000 cc

55. How should you estimate the amount of blood loss?

    a. Pour a pint of fluid on the floor and soak a garment in it.
    b. Wait for signs of hypoperfusion to appear.
    c. Remove the patient's clothing.
    d. Ask the patient.

56. What is the first line of treatment for this patient?

    a. Ensure an open airway.
    b. Obtain a detailed history.
    c. Wait for signs of hypoperfusion to appear.
    d. Administer CPR.

57. Which of the following steps is NOT considered standard operating procedure for using an AED?

    a. For an unwitnessed cardiac arrest, perform five cycles of CPR, and then apply the AED.
    b. For a witnessed cardiac arrest in an adult, apply the AED immediately.
    c. Continue to apply shocks until the pulse is regained but alternate with cycles of CPR.
    d. Apply two shocks, and then wait for the AED to provide a message on how to proceed.

58. You enter the home of the mother of an 18-month-old baby. She frantically recounts that she stepped out of the bathroom for a phone call. Upon her return, the baby was submerged and blue. What is your first action?

    a. Assess the baby for pulse and respirations; if applicable, begin CPR.
    b. Report the mother for child endangerment.
    c. Apply oxygen and transport the baby.
    d. Wrap the baby in warm blankets and transport.

59. You are responding to a 911 call for an elderly woman who has fallen. When you enter the home, a family member who cares for the patient leads you to her bedroom. As you begin to examine the patient, you notice old bruises all over her body, and it looks as though she has had black eyes recently. You notice she seems reluctant to talk to you and continues to glance over at the family member present in the room. What do you note as part of your evaluation?

    a. The patient appears to be clumsy
    b. Possible prescription medication abuse
    c. Possible need for long-term care placement
    d. Possible elder abuse

60. You arrive on the scene to treat a child who is having difficulty breathing. The mother is crying and appears hysterical. What is the best course of action?

    a. Try to reassure the mother, ask her to breathe deeply to calm down, and explain that the child will respond better to treatment if the parents are calm.

    b. Ask the mother to leave the room until she calms down.

    c. Offer a sedative to help the mother calm down.

    d. Tell the mother sternly to stop crying.

61. Which arteries do you use to assess the pulses of an infant?

    a. Brachial and temporal arteries

    b. Brachial and femoral arteries

    c. Carotid and femoral arteries

    d. Carotid and temporal arteries

62. You receive a call from a young woman whose car has been struck in a shopping mall parking lot. She is concerned about the elderly man who backed into her car. On arrival at the scene, you find a conscious 88-year-old man who appears to be having an acute ischemic stroke. What would be the most appropriate course of action?

    a. Perform a physical exam.

    b. Administer oxygen and obtain a patient history.

    c. Monitor blood pressure.

    d. Administer oxygen and provide transport to the hospital for fibrinolytic therapy.

63. How can you determine if a laceration involves an artery or a vein?

    a. A vein bleeds bright red blood with high pressure.

    b. A vein bleeds dark red blood, steadily, but with low pressure.

    c. An artery bleeds bright red blood, with low pressure.

    d. A vein oozes slowly.

64. As an EMT, which of the following is NOT a typical step when dealing with a potential fire situation at the scene of a car accident?

    a. Grab a fire extinguisher, and try to put out the fire.

    b. Turn off the car ignition if the car is still running.

    c. Ask bystanders to refrain from smoking.

    d. Survey the scene to check for downed wires or fluid leakage from the car.

65. You respond to a 911 call for a possible gunshot wound patient. You arrive before the police and notice an injured man lying on the street with several men arguing in his vicinity. Which *initial* action is preferable?

    a. Instruct the men to leave so you can treat the patient.

    b. Wait for the police to secure the scene, and then proceed.

    c. Explain to the bystanders that the police are on their way, and then proceed.

    d. Drive slowly into the crowd so you can access the injured person.

66. The baby's head is crowning, and you begin to prepare for imminent delivery. Which of the following would NOT be an appropriate action during delivery?

a. Set up a sterile field using sterile towels or paper barriers.
b. Loosen the umbilical cord if it is wrapped around the baby's neck.
c. Carefully break the amniotic sac if it is still intact.
d. Press gently on the fontanelles in order to prevent tearing of the perineum.

67. All of the following are basic supplies that all ambulances should be equipped with EXCEPT:

a. Ballistic vests
b. Suction equipment
c. Splinting supplies
d. AED

68. Signs of respiratory arrest in an infant differ from those of an adult. Which of the following signs indicate respiratory arrest in an infant?

a. Breathing rate less than 15 breaths per minute, slow heart rate
b. Breathing rate less than 10 breaths per minute, slow heart rate
c. Breathing rate less than 20 breaths per minute, fast heart rate
d. Breathing rate less than 30 breaths per minute, slow heart rate

69. How should chemical burns to the eyes should be treated?

a. Flush with vinegar or baking soda.
b. Cover the eye with a moistened pad.
c. Flood the eye with water for at least 20 minutes.
d. Cover the eye and transporting the patient.

70. Which of the following statements regarding use of the ambulance siren is FALSE?

a. Use the siren when close to the vehicle ahead of you to alert the driver.
b. Continuous use of a siren can increase an operator's driving speed.
c. Use of a siren can make motorists less inclined to give the right of way.
d. Use of a siren can worsen the condition of a patient.

71. You respond to a call for a nine-year-old with a possible fractured arm. As you approach the house, you realize that you have been on multiple calls to this address. Your assessment of the child reveals small burns and multiple bruises in various stages of healing, in addition to the deformity of the arm. The child is quiet and withdrawn. What is your response?

a. Accuse the parents of child abuse and then transport the child for treatment.
b. Transport the child, and report your suspicions to your supervisor for notification of the proper agency.
c. Transport the child for treatment, and then call the police.
d. Write your report, including your opinion about the abuse.

72. When a patient has an open abdominal wound with evisceration, what type of dressing do you apply?
   a. Dry sterile gauze, covered with Vaseline gauze, then a compression dressing
   b. Sterile gauze, moistened with sterile saline or water, covered with Vaseline gauze (occlusive)
   c. Replace organs into the abdomen, then apply Vaseline gauze
   d. Sterile bulky dressing to keep wound from further eviscerating

73. Which of the following is NOT a recommended action when responding to an emergency call that is also a possible crime scene?
   a. Wait for the police to arrive.
   b. Be careful when entering the scene so potential evidence is not disturbed.
   c. Document the reason for any delay in treatment.
   d. Enter the scene immediately to begin emergency medical treatment for the patient.

74. In what cases is use of the PASG indicated?
   a. Cardiogenic shock
   b. Shock in the presence of a chest wound
   c. Pelvic injury
   d. Congestive heart failure

75. What is an example of a medical condition that can mimic a psychiatric condition?
   a. Heart attack
   b. Diabetes
   c. Asthma
   d. Allergic reaction

76. What is the problem in the case of an infiltrated IV?
   a. The IV fluid flows into surrounding tissue.
   b. The IV flow rate is too fast.
   c. Tubing is caught under the backboard.
   d. Tubing has pulled out of the catheter.

77. All of the following are considerations for possible inhaled toxins EXCEPT:
   a. Inhaled toxins can cause difficulty breathing and airway swelling.
   b. Inhaled toxins are not as quickly absorbed; therefore, the consequences are not as great as with ingested toxins.
   c. Inhaled toxins can be present in the air and may affect others in the immediate area.
   d. Inhaled toxins can cause fainting or seizures.

78. When you inspect the feet of a homeless man after exposure to extremely cold temperatures, you observe that the skin of his toes is white and waxy and feels frozen on palpitation. What do you suspect?
   a. Superficial injury
   b. Shock
   c. Good prognosis
   d. Deep-tissue damage

Answer Key and Explanations for Test #2

1. D: Children or mentally incompetent adults cannot legally refuse treatment. Care can be given to a child without parental consent in the case of life-threatening illness or injury when the parent or guardian is not present.

2. C: The initial treatment for epistaxis is the application of pressure (pinching) to the nostrils, because most nosebleeds originate in the anterior portion of the nose. Lean the patient forward to prevent blood from going down the throat. Do not have the patient lie back in the Trendelenburg position; the increased blood pressure to the head would exacerbate the bleeding. Keep the patient calm and quiet to decrease the blood pressure. If the nosebleed does not stop with applied pressure, the patient may need nasal packing in the ER.

3. B: It is extremely important to note that even in the absence of pain, a spinal injury may still be present. Any potential spinal cord injury should be immobilized immediately. The patient should be instructed to try not to move at all. When questioning the patient, it is important to position yourself in a way that allows him to see you without turning his head. Important information to gain from the patient may include describing any pain, tenderness, or tingling they may be feeling, exactly what happened in the circumstances surrounding the injury, ability to move the fingers and toes, and also to ask him if he is able to tell where you are touching him at the moment. You may ask the patient to grab both your hands and squeeze in order to assess the equality of the strength in each hand. If the patient is unable to respond, document any important details about the accident scene, such as where the patient was located and the position they were found in.

4. D: Advanced airway techniques can expose an EMT to a number of potential infectious diseases, such as HIV or hepatitis, through contact with bodily fluids. To help prevent this from occurring, a mask, eye protection, and gloves should be worn. Before the tube is inserted, the cuff must be checked for air leaks by inflating the cuff then gently squeezing while listening for air escaping. Tubes come in a range of sizes. Most men will need an 8 to 8.5 mm tube, while women will likely need 7 to 8 mm. Having a 7.5 mm tube on hand will cover most all emergencies. A stylus should be placed into the tube to help with placement, because the tube is flexible and it will be difficult to control the tip of the tube without the support of the stylus.

5. C: A blood glucose level of 80 mg/dL or lower indicates hypoglycemia, or low blood glucose. A normal reading for blood glucose level is 80 to 120 mg/dL. Hyperglycemia is an extremely high glucose level. Diabetes is the general term for the medical condition that prevents insulin production or effective metabolism.

6. B: Other conditions such as diabetes, epilepsy, and hypoxia may also produce symptoms resembling those of alcohol intoxication. Given that the patient has hit his head, his symptoms could be due to head injury.

7. A: Because intoxicated patients could also be suffering from a medical emergency or an injury, they should be transported to the hospital for further assessment. Patients with even minor head injuries may be prone to subdural hematoma. Asking the patient if he has taken drugs may provoke a violent reaction, and calling law enforcement without properly assessing the patient's condition may result in serious adverse events or even death.

8. C: Substance or alcohol abusers may appear calm and then suddenly become violent. For your own protection, if the situation becomes unsafe and you have not been trained in law enforcement, you should immediately leave the scene and call the police for assistance.

9. B: Four-way flashers or directional signals should not be used as emergency lights because they can confuse other drivers.

10. D: A scrape where the top layers of the skin are missing is an abrasion. A contusion is a bruise. A puncture is a wound that is deep and narrow. A laceration refers to a cut in the skin usually caused by a sharp object.

11. D: Although burns caused by electrical current may result in relatively minor skin injury, they can present a high risk of severe internal injury.

12. C: Labor consists of three stages. The first stage starts with contractions that help to propel the baby closer to the birth canal. Initially, the contractions can be abnormal and far apart, but as labor progresses, the contractions will be closer together. The cervix dilates and is measured in centimeters to gauge how far along the first stage of labor is. Contractions help to prepare the cervix, and the presence of bloody show can be seen during this phase. Ten centimeters is the dilation needed to attain in order for the baby's head to fit through the birth canal. A woman enters the second stage of labor as the baby's head enters the birth canal and can be seen through the vaginal opening. This is known as crowning. When this is observed, it is an indication that the baby will be born very quickly and on the scene. The third stage of labor is the afterbirth where the placenta is delivered.

13. C: The most frequently seen symptom of respiratory distress is a change in the respiratory rate, either faster or slower. Cyanosis is a bluish cast of the skin and mucous membranes because of a low oxygen level. Absent respiratory sounds indicate respiratory failure. A change in consciousness may occur because of an inadequate level of oxygen to the brain, but it would not be the most commonly observed symptom of acute respiratory distress.

14. C: Hypoglycemia means low blood sugar or a blood sugar reading that is less than 70 mg/dL. This happens when too much insulin is in the blood or too little glucose is available. If a person has diabetes, hypoglycemia can occur if a meal is skipped, during illness, or from an increase in exercise without increasing food intake. Symptoms of hypoglycemia can include sweating, hunger, headache, rapid heartbeat, irritability, confusion, or disorientation. Hypoglycemia can progress into seizures, convulsions, fainting, or a coma. It is important to recognize symptoms of hypoglycemia. It may not always be known if someone being treated has diabetes, and the patient may not be wearing a Medic Alert bracelet. Hyperglycemia means high blood sugar. The symptoms of hyperglycemia are frequent urination, increased thirst and hunger, weight loss, tingling in the feet, cuts that don't heal well, feeling tired, and sugar in the urine. The blood glucose level is typically greater than 180 mg/dL.

15. C: As the patient is being examined for possible injuries, the acronym that is helpful to remember is DCAP-BTLS. This stands for deformity, contusions, abrasion, punctures or penetrations, burns, tenderness, lacerations, and swelling. Each area of the body is examined, typically starting with the head and moving downward to the neck, chest, abdominal region, and lower extremities. This rapid trauma assessment should only take about one to two minutes of your time. If an injury is identified as the assessment is under way, another EMS should address that injury while the trauma assessment is completed.

16. B: The best line of treatment for a child with diarrhea and vomiting is to maintain an open airway and administer oxygen. Oral suctioning may be required for vomiting. Sipping water or ice chips is usually recommended for children with diarrhea only.

17. C: The first step in assessing a child with fever is to obtain a relative skin temperature using a skin thermometer or by applying the back of your hand to the child's forehead or abdomen. Oral or rectal temperatures are generally not taken in the prehospital setting.

18. A: If a child has a seizure on transport, you should maintain an open airway and administer oxygen. Never insert an oropharyngeal airway or a bite stick. Seizures caused by fever should always be considered life-threatening.

19. D: Activated charcoal is contraindicated in patients who have ingested acids or alkalis, such as those found in bathroom or oven cleaners, in patients who have ingested gasoline during siphoning, and in those with altered mental status.

20. C: In a twin birth, the placenta may deliver either before or after the birth of the second twin. There may be a separate placenta for each baby or a single one for both. Breech birth is common in the second twin; the umbilical cord of the first twin should be tied or cut before the birth of the second twin.

21. C: The avulsed body part should be saved by wrapping it in a dry sterile dressing and then placing it in a plastic bag, plastic wrap, or aluminum foil. Do not place the part in dry ice, water, or saline.

22. D: The best method of care for an open abdominal injury is to apply a sterile saline dressing over the wound, then apply an occlusive dressing. Never give the patient something by mouth or touch, or replace an exposed or eviscerated organ. Use of an aluminum foil occlusive dressing may cut an eviscerated organ.

23. D: He likely sustained a closed crush injury. This type of injury occurs when extreme force is placed on an area of the body. The injury is inside and does not openly bleed externally. There may be internal bleeding, and shock is a possibility. An open crush injury would involve soft tissue damage and possible damage to internal organs. The wound is open and can be seen with the eye. A laceration is a cut in the skin. The width and depth can vary. An abrasion is a type of scrape that occurs that typically involves the epidermal layer of skin. The wound is superficial but can be very painful. A contusion is another term for a bruise where there is damage to the soft tissue. An avulsion is when part of the tissue is torn off the body. An amputation is when a body part is physically separated from the body. Massive bleeding may occur in the setting of an accidental amputation.

24. B: All aspects of patient care are considered confidential. This means that the patient has the right to privacy, even if other people are around who are not directly authorized to provide care to the patient. An EMT must be sensitive to this information and not discuss any private information in front of others. The patient must give permission for information to be given to others. There are exceptions to this rule. When the patient's care is being transferred from the EMS to the hospital, information must be reported. There are many incidents that require police assistance, and information can be divulged in these cases. These include cases of rape, abuse, accidents occurring in the workplace, gunshot wounds, or animal bites. Information can be provided to insurance companies in order for payment to be received, and information can be discussed in court if an EMT is subpoenaed. Care should not be discussed with a neighbor, the media, or anyone else who is not authorized.

25. C: Remove the patient from the water after placing him on a long backboard and securing his head with a cervical spine immobilization device or with manual stabilization of the head.

26. A: Anaphylaxis is the term used for a severe allergic reaction.

27. B: After donning protective gloves, assure that the patient has an open airway and ventilation, and then address the laceration by applying concentrated direct pressure. Apply a tourniquet only if directed to do so by a physician. If the patient is in cardiac arrest, then CPR is appropriate.

28. A: If previously prescribed for the patient, the EMT may assist him or her in taking nitroglycerin, epinephrine, or inhalers. Permission from medical direction may be required.

29. A: This child has a critical burn, so you establish an airway and transport him immediately. You can perform all other treatments en route.

30. C: In a child, the tongue is larger, the chest wall is softer, and the trachea is narrower compared with those of an adult.

31. B: The signs and symptoms of carbon monoxide poisoning may resemble those of the flu, including nausea and headache.

32. D: The jaw-thrust maneuver is the only recommended procedure for opening the airway in an unconscious patient with a possible spinal injury.

33. D: Oxygen should never be withheld from a patient in respiratory distress, even those with a chronic lung disease, such as bronchitis or emphysema.

34. B: Typical body changes during the last trimester include increases in heart rate, blood volume, and cardiac output. Blood pressure usually decreases slightly.

35. C: Rapid trauma assessment is indicated in patients with significant mechanisms of injury, such as penetrating wounds to the head, neck, chest, or abdomen, falls from a height of >15 feet (such as from a tall building), or multiple long bone fractures.

36. A: A typical nitroglycerin dose will be 0.3 to 0.4 milligrams (mg). It is available as a sublingual (under the tongue) tablet, spray, or extended-release capsule. A prescription for extended-release capsules can usually be taken orally three to four times per day. Nitroglycerin given via spray or tablet is usually taken on an as-needed or PRN basis and can be taken up to 10 minutes before any activity that will likely cause angina to occur. If medical authorization has been obtained to give a patient nitroglycerin, the expiration date should be verified before giving a dose. Once the bottle has been opened, nitroglycerin tablets will lose their potency once they have been exposed to light and thus may not be as effective. If no prescription is available, talk with the physician to see if an order is indicated. The patient needs to be properly positioned in a sitting or lying position in case hypotension occurs. Vital signs should be monitored after each dose. An EMT may typically assist with up to three doses given three to five minutes apart as needed.

37. B: In the case of a near-drowning, rescue breathing should be initiated without delay, even if the victim is still in the water. Chest compression is only effective when the victim is out of the water.

38. D: Do not attempt to collect a venomous snake or spider for identification.

39. C: In a young child with possible airway obstruction, attempts to remove a mild obstruction may result in severe obstruction. Back blows and chest thrusts should only be performed in the case of a severe obstruction, and finger sweeps should only be performed when the child is unconscious and the object is visible in the mouth. The most appropriate course of action is to avoid agitating the child and provide immediate transport to the hospital.

40. A: Young children typically fear a stranger in their environment and will maintain eye contact with that person. Thus, inattentiveness to your presence is indicative of an altered mental state.

41. D: High fever, generalized rash, and altered mental state are indicative of meningitis, or inflammation of the tissue protecting the brain and spinal cord. Because a child with meningitis is at high risk for seizures, his or her condition should be carefully monitored during transport to the hospital.

42. C: A child loses blood at the same rate as an adult, so the same wound can be much more serious in a child.

43. C: If the baby is in rigor mortis, do not attempt resuscitation. Observe the scene details, and document it carefully. Comfort the parents, and then contact your medical base to determine transfer protocol.

44. B: A bronchodilator is a type of medication that is administered via an inhaler and is administered directly into the lungs through inhalation. This type of medication is called a beta antagonist bronchodilator and helps the bronchioles to dilate or open up in order to improve oxygen exchange. Generic forms of bronchodilators are albuterol, metaproterenol, and isoetharine. Brand names of bronchodilators include Alupent, Proventil, Metaprel, Ventolin, Bronkosol, Brovana, and Foradil. Pulmicort is a type of inhaled steroid that acts as an anti-inflammatory. These are typically prescribed if a patient is using a bronchodilator more than twice a week or if the patient's asthma interferes with normal activities. Other types of inhaled steroids include AeroBid, Flovent, Azmacort, and Alvesco.

45. D: "Coffee-ground" emesis is the classic sign of bleeding from the stomach. Bleeding from the colon may be red or black and tarry in appearance. Hematuria is the term for bleeding from the bladder, which causes the urine to appear pink. Hemoptysis refers to bloodstained sputum from the respiratory system.

46. B: The general rule of thumb for establishing the FiO_2 (fraction of inspired oxygen) is to begin with a baseline of 20% for regular breathing air, and then add 4% for each 1 L/min above that. In this case, 20% + (5 L/min × 4%) = 40%.

47. A: Oxygen tanks contain gas under very high pressure and may explode if ruptured. Always handle these tanks with care, and store in a manner that prevents movement when transporting. Wrapping the tanks with blankets is not a necessary precaution, but securing the tanks to prevent rolling or falling is essential. The valves and gauges are the most fragile parts of the tank, and they require extra care when transporting.

48. B: The boy is loudly wheezing and has facial edema; both of these signs indicate a severe allergic reaction. Because the boy's physician ordered the epinephrine autoinjector pen, call for medical direction and then administer the medication. The child is already having signs of respiratory distress, and without intervention he may progress into full anaphylactic shock. The child may know how to give himself the injection, but because he is already having difficulty breathing, the better choice would be to get medical direction, then administer the drug.

49. B: Use room-temperature sterile water or saline to stop the burning process. Cover the burn with a clean, dry dressing. Do not apply ointments, lotions, or antiseptics, and avoid opening any blisters. Keep the patient warm during transport.

50. B: If air is escaping through the nose and mouth, the immediate action is to close the mouth and pinch the nose.

51. A: A patient with an injury to the tibia or fibula should be treated for shock. Administer high-concentration oxygen and splint the injury. Do not apply manual traction or tension and do not apply an ice pack directly to the skin.

52. B: There are two types of devices available for establishing and maintaining an airway. The oropharyngeal airway goes into the patient's mouth and helps keep the tongue in the proper position to prevent obstruction. This type of airway may stimulate the gag reflex, which can cause vomiting to occur. This would place the patient at risk for aspiration. If the patient is unconscious, the gag reflex will not be present and this airway can be used. The nasopharyngeal airway utilizes a flexible tube that is inserted through the patient's nostril to establish an airway. This type of airway is less likely to stimulate the gag reflex and is therefore a safer choice for a conscious patient having trouble keeping their airway open. This is also the airway of choice for anyone who is in the active stage of a seizure.

53. D: The zygomatic arch is the formation that consists of a slender bar of bone found on each side of the face that connects the cheekbone to the temporal bone. Mandible is the medical term for the lower jawbone. Maxilla is the pair of bones that fuses at the midline to form the upper jawbone. The orbit is the round cavity in the skull in which the eye is located.

54. D: In an adult, sudden blood loss of 1,000 cc, or 1 liter, is considered serious; however, because children have a lower blood volume compared with adults, blood loss of 500 cc is considered serious in a child. Blood loss of 150 cc would be serious in an infant.

55. A: Although it is difficult to estimate blood loss, a useful method is to pour a pint of liquid on the floor and soak a garment in it to observe how wet it looks and feels. In a patient with blood loss, do not wait for signs of hypoperfusion or shock to develop to begin treatment.

56. A: In this case, bleeding from the rectum is a sign of internal bleeding, which may rapidly lead to hypoperfusion or shock. In cases of suspected internal bleeding, the first step should be to ensure an open airway and assess breathing and circulation. Do not wait for signs of shock to appear before beginning treatment.

57. C: The AED can be used immediately if the cardiac arrest was witnessed. An unwitnessed cardiac arrest requires the use of five cycles of CPR, which is approximately two minutes in length. Once the CPR cycles are completed, the AED should be applied. All direct contact with the patient should be stopped while the AED is in use. Shocking should not be continuously applied until a pulse rate is regained. Rather, shocks should be delivered, then the message from the AED should be noted and may indicate that no shock should be delivered. If additional shocks are needed, authorization should be obtained from the physician.

58. A: Because the baby is cyanotic, it is probable that it has no respirations or pulse. Assess the vital signs and if applicable, start CPR. The mother may be guilty of child neglect; the ER physicians may choose to report her to authorities, but at this point, the child is in a life-threatening situation and needs immediate intervention. Administer CPR first to attempt to revive the child. All other treatments, such as warm blankets, are secondary to reestablishing a pulse and respirations.

59. D: There are potential signs of elder abuse. There are three types of elder abuse—domestic, institutional, and self-neglect. Domestic abuse is maltreatment of an elderly person by the caregiver. Abuse can be physical, sexual, psychological, or in the form of neglect by either the person or the caregiver. It can also involve financial exploitation. Signs of physical abuse in an elderly person may include evidence of injuries in various states of healing, fractures, wounds, or indications that the person has been restrained. Laboratory tests may reveal excessive drug levels or the absence of prescribed drugs in the system. The caregiver may often refuse to leave the patient alone with medical personnel. If any form of abuse is suspected, it is imperative to report it to Elder Protective Services. Laws vary from state to state, but EMS are generally mandated to report such issues.

60. A: It is very likely that when an EMT is responding to a situation involving a child, the parents or family will react emotionally. It is important to remember that a professional and caring demeanor must be maintained at all times while trying to treat the child. Any interaction with the family should be calm and supportive. A rule of thumb to remember is that if the parents remain calm, the child will likely remain calm. If the parents are agitated or hysterical, the child may react the same way. Help to calm the parents' anxiety by explaining what is happening and provide reassurance. It is important to refrain from making any promises to the parents about whether their child will be alright. Providing tips on calming down, such as deep breathing, can be helpful. Parents can be useful in administering oxygen and helping to keep the child calm, but it is important to remember not to separate the child from the parents or family unless medically necessary.

61. B: Assess the pulse of an infant by palpating the brachial or femoral arteries.

62. D: In patients with acute ischemic stroke, administering oxygen is the most important first step, followed by rapid transport to the hospital for fibrinolytic therapy. Fibrinolytic therapy must be performed within 3 hours of symptom onset.

63. B: A lacerated vein steadily bleeds dark red blood. An artery bleeds rapidly, and the blood is bright red.

64. A: The risk of fire is inherent in many accident-type situations involving motor vehicles, hazardous products, electric wires, and other factors. Extinguishing a fire should only be attempted if specialized training has been received. When an EMT arrives on the scene, the area should be surveyed to check for potentially dangerous situations, such as downed power lines or fluids leaking from a car. If a car is noted to be running, the ignition should be turned off. Smoking anywhere in the area should be avoided. Downed power lines should also be avoided due to the risk of electric shock or death. If there is a person inside a car around downed power lines, the person should remain where they are until the power lines have been disconnected.

65. B: The presence of arguing men indicates the possibility of personal injury to you. Wait for the police to secure the scene prior to proceeding to assess the injured man.

66. D: If it appears likely that a baby is going to be born imminently without time to get to the hospital, there are steps to take to get ready for the birth. First, all precautions should be taken to avoid contact with any bodily fluid. Next, a sterile field should be set up, utilizing sterile towels or a sterile paper barrier around the lower part of the woman's body. As crowning occurs, it is important NOT to press on the baby's fontanelles, as this is the area that allows for brain growth during the infant's first year. The amniotic sac should be punctured if it is still intact at this point in the delivery. It is extremely important to look at the position of the umbilical cord. If it is wrapped around the baby's neck, attempts should be made to loosen and remove it prior to delivery. If this is not possible, clamp the cord in two places, and then cut the cord to remove the danger.

67. A: Rules and regulations vary from state to state and also within the local jurisdiction as to what is stocked on an ambulance for medical supplies. Nonmedical supplies also vary. Personal protective equipment is mandated though to help prevent EMS personnel from acquiring communicable diseases. This type of equipment includes gowns, masks, gloves, and eyewear. Ballistic vests are sometimes worn by EMS personnel who may work in more violent or dangerous areas, but use of these vests is usually personal preference. Medical supplies that are usually included on an ambulance are suctioning equipment, splinting supplies, first-aid materials for caring for wounds, childbirth supplies, and a variety of medications including epinephrine, nitroglycerin, and albuterol sulfate. Supplies needed to ventilate the patient are always stocked, along with an automated external defibrillator and cardiac compression equipment. Nonmedical supplies may include binoculars, maps, and emergency routes that have been preplanned for efficiency.

68. B: Signs of respiratory arrest in an infant include a breathing rate of less than 10 breaths per minute, limp muscle tone, unresponsive, slow or absent heart rate, and weak or absent pulse.

69. C: In treating a chemical burn to the eye, immediately flood the eye with water; continue washing the eye during transport for at least 20 minutes or until arrival at the hospital. Do not use vinegar or baking soda to neutralize the chemical.

70. A: Sounding the siren when close to another vehicle can result in the driver panicking and jamming on his brakes; use the horn to alert the driver instead. Continuous use of a siren can make motorists less likely to yield the right of way, can increase stress and anxiety in injured or ill patients, and has been associated with increased operator driving speed.

71. B: Your main objective is the treatment of the child. Report the suspected abuse to your supervisor. Record the injuries and factual information regarding the child's environment and any comments made by the parents or caregivers in quotes, keep a copy for yourself, and give a copy to your supervisor to present to the proper authorities.

72. B: The proper dressing for a wound with evisceration of internal organs is sterile gauze, moistened with sterile water or saline to keep the viscera from becoming dry. Place an occlusive dressing, such as Vaseline gauze, over the sterile moistened gauze, to maintain the moisture content. Never attempt to replace the organs into the abdomen. Position the patient with the knees flexed, if not contraindicated by a spinal injury, to prevent stretching of the abdominal muscles and further evisceration. Dry dressings would adhere to the viscera. Bulky dressings would apply pressure and possibly force the viscera back into the abdominal cavity, increasing the risk of infection.

73. D: Oftentimes when an emergency call is made, the scene is also identified as a possible crime scene. The first and foremost concern is EMT safety. The next concern is the emergency treatment of the patient. The EMT should not enter a crime scene unless police have arrived on the scene. Any delays that occur in treating the patient, such as having to wait for police, should be carefully documented. The EMT must take care not to interfere with the crime scene or disturb evidence. The exception would be if the potential evidence is interfering with the emergency treatment of the patient. In the case of a gunshot wound, it is important to try not to destroy the clothing when removing it from the patient, as this may be an important piece of evidence. Documentation of anything the EMT has seen or heard while at the scene is also very important. Any information documented should be objective and factual.

74. C: The pneumatic anti-shock garment (PASG) is indicated in cases of bleeding, pelvic injury, or abdominal trauma. It is contraindicated in patients with cardiogenic shock or shock in the presence of a chest wound.

75. B: Diabetes or low blood sugar can produce symptoms—such as hostile behavior, drooling, heavy perspiration, or seizures—that mimic those of a psychiatric condition.

76. A: In the case of an infiltrated IV, the needle has either punctured the vein and exited the other side or pulled out of the vein entirely, resulting in fluid flowing into the surrounding tissue. The IV flow should be stopped, and the IV should be discontinued.

77. B: Inhaled toxins can be very dangerous. Because the toxins enter the body through the lungs, absorption is very quick and can lead to poisoning throughout the body. The lining of the airway can be burned by the toxins, and this can lead to difficulty breathing, coughing, and closing of the throat due to swelling. Effects can also include headaches, feeling dizzy, fainting, seizures, and changed mental status. When you encounter a situation that involves inhaled toxins, you immediately should be concerned with potential effects on others in the area. The poison or toxin can still be present in the air. In the case of carbon monoxide, it will not be able to be detected, since it is colorless and odorless. If training has been completed on the use of a self-contained breathing apparatus (SCBA), this should immediately be employed. Otherwise, you will need to wait for specially trained responders. The main goal in initial treatment is to prevent a quick deterioration. The airway should be established and oxygen administered.

78. D: Deep-tissue damage from exposure to cold presents with signs and symptoms of white, waxy skin; firm or frozen feel upon palpation; possible swelling or blisters; lack of feeling; and, if it is thawed, the skin appears flushed, red or purple, mottled, pale, or cyanotic.

EMT Practice Tests #3, #4, and #5

To take these additional EMT practice tests, visit our bonus page:
mometrix.com/bonus948/emt

How to Overcome Test Anxiety

Just the thought of taking a test is enough to make most people a little nervous. A test is an important event that can have a long-term impact on your future, so it's important to take it seriously and it's natural to feel anxious about performing well. But just because anxiety is normal, that doesn't mean that it's helpful in test taking, or that you should simply accept it as part of your life. Anxiety can have a variety of effects. These effects can be mild, like making you feel slightly nervous, or severe, like blocking your ability to focus or remember even a simple detail.

If you experience test anxiety—whether severe or mild—it's important to know how to beat it. To discover this, first you need to understand what causes test anxiety.

Causes of Test Anxiety

While we often think of anxiety as an uncontrollable emotional state, it can actually be caused by simple, practical things. One of the most common causes of test anxiety is that a person does not feel adequately prepared for their test. This feeling can be the result of many different issues such as poor study habits or lack of organization, but the most common culprit is time management. Starting to study too late, failing to organize your study time to cover all of the material, or being distracted while you study will mean that you're not well prepared for the test. This may lead to cramming the night before, which will cause you to be physically and mentally exhausted for the test. Poor time management also contributes to feelings of stress, fear, and hopelessness as you realize you are not well prepared but don't know what to do about it.

Other times, test anxiety is not related to your preparation for the test but comes from unresolved fear. This may be a past failure on a test, or poor performance on tests in general. It may come from comparing yourself to others who seem to be performing better or from the stress of living up to expectations. Anxiety may be driven by fears of the future—how failure on this test would affect your educational and career goals. These fears are often completely irrational, but they can still negatively impact your test performance.

Elements of Test Anxiety

As mentioned earlier, test anxiety is considered to be an emotional state, but it has physical and mental components as well. Sometimes you may not even realize that you are suffering from test anxiety until you notice the physical symptoms. These can include trembling hands, rapid heartbeat, sweating, nausea, and tense muscles. Extreme anxiety may lead to fainting or vomiting. Obviously, any of these symptoms can have a negative impact on testing. It is important to recognize them as soon as they begin to occur so that you can address the problem before it damages your performance.

The mental components of test anxiety include trouble focusing and inability to remember learned information. During a test, your mind is on high alert, which can help you recall information and stay focused for an extended period of time. However, anxiety interferes with your mind's natural processes, causing you to blank out, even on the questions you know well. The strain of testing during anxiety makes it difficult to stay focused, especially on a test that may take several hours. Extreme anxiety can take a huge mental toll, making it difficult not only to recall test information but even to understand the test questions or pull your thoughts together.

233

Effects of Test Anxiety

Test anxiety is like a disease—if left untreated, it will get progressively worse. Anxiety leads to poor performance, and this reinforces the feelings of fear and failure, which in turn lead to poor performances on subsequent tests. It can grow from a mild nervousness to a crippling condition. If allowed to progress, test anxiety can have a big impact on your schooling, and consequently on your future.

Test anxiety can spread to other parts of your life. Anxiety on tests can become anxiety in any stressful situation, and blanking on a test can turn into panicking in a job situation. But fortunately, you don't have to let anxiety rule your testing and determine your grades. There are a number of relatively simple steps you can take to move past anxiety and function normally on a test and in the rest of life.

Physical Steps for Beating Test Anxiety

While test anxiety is a serious problem, the good news is that it can be overcome. It doesn't have to control your ability to think and remember information. While it may take time, you can begin taking steps today to beat anxiety.

Just as your first hint that you may be struggling with anxiety comes from the physical symptoms, the first step to treating it is also physical. Rest is crucial for having a clear, strong mind. If you are tired, it is much easier to give in to anxiety. But if you establish good sleep habits, your body and mind will be ready to perform optimally, without the strain of exhaustion. Additionally, sleeping well helps you to retain information better, so you're more likely to recall the answers when you see the test questions.

Getting good sleep means more than going to bed on time. It's important to allow your brain time to relax. Take study breaks from time to time so it doesn't get overworked, and don't study right before bed. Take time to rest your mind before trying to rest your body, or you may find it difficult to fall asleep.

Along with sleep, other aspects of physical health are important in preparing for a test. Good nutrition is vital for good brain function. Sugary foods and drinks may give a burst of energy but this burst is followed by a crash, both physically and emotionally. Instead, fuel your body with protein and vitamin-rich foods.

Also, drink plenty of water. Dehydration can lead to headaches and exhaustion, especially if your brain is already under stress from the rigors of the test. Particularly if your test is a long one, drink water during the breaks. And if possible, take an energy-boosting snack to eat between sections.

Along with sleep and diet, a third important part of physical health is exercise. Maintaining a steady workout schedule is helpful, but even taking 5-minute study breaks to walk can help get your blood pumping faster and clear your head. Exercise also releases endorphins, which contribute to a positive feeling and can help combat test anxiety.

When you nurture your physical health, you are also contributing to your mental health. If your body is healthy, your mind is much more likely to be healthy as well. So take time to rest, nourish your body with healthy food and water, and get moving as much as possible. Taking these physical steps will make you stronger and more able to take the mental steps necessary to overcome test anxiety.

Mental Steps for Beating Test Anxiety

Working on the mental side of test anxiety can be more challenging, but as with the physical side, there are clear steps you can take to overcome it. As mentioned earlier, test anxiety often stems from lack of preparation, so the obvious solution is to prepare for the test. Effective studying may be the most important weapon you have for beating test anxiety, but you can and should employ several other mental tools to combat fear.

First, boost your confidence by reminding yourself of past success—tests or projects that you aced. If you're putting as much effort into preparing for this test as you did for those, there's no reason you should expect to fail here. Work hard to prepare; then trust your preparation.

Second, surround yourself with encouraging people. It can be helpful to find a study group, but be sure that the people you're around will encourage a positive attitude. If you spend time with others who are anxious or cynical, this will only contribute to your own anxiety. Look for others who are motivated to study hard from a desire to succeed, not from a fear of failure.

Third, reward yourself. A test is physically and mentally tiring, even without anxiety, and it can be helpful to have something to look forward to. Plan an activity following the test, regardless of the outcome, such as going to a movie or getting ice cream.

When you are taking the test, if you find yourself beginning to feel anxious, remind yourself that you know the material. Visualize successfully completing the test. Then take a few deep, relaxing breaths and return to it. Work through the questions carefully but with confidence, knowing that you are capable of succeeding.

Developing a healthy mental approach to test taking will also aid in other areas of life. Test anxiety affects more than just the actual test—it can be damaging to your mental health and even contribute to depression. It's important to beat test anxiety before it becomes a problem for more than testing.

Study Strategy

Being prepared for the test is necessary to combat anxiety, but what does being prepared look like? You may study for hours on end and still not feel prepared. What you need is a strategy for test prep. The next few pages outline our recommended steps to help you plan out and conquer the challenge of preparation.

STEP 1: SCOPE OUT THE TEST

Learn everything you can about the format (multiple choice, essay, etc.) and what will be on the test. Gather any study materials, course outlines, or sample exams that may be available. Not only will this help you to prepare, but knowing what to expect can help to alleviate test anxiety.

STEP 2: MAP OUT THE MATERIAL

Look through the textbook or study guide and make note of how many chapters or sections it has. Then divide these over the time you have. For example, if a book has 15 chapters and you have five days to study, you need to cover three chapters each day. Even better, if you have the time, leave an extra day at the end for overall review after you have gone through the material in depth.

If time is limited, you may need to prioritize the material. Look through it and make note of which sections you think you already have a good grasp on, and which need review. While you are studying, skim quickly through the familiar sections and take more time on the challenging parts.

Write out your plan so you don't get lost as you go. Having a written plan also helps you feel more in control of the study, so anxiety is less likely to arise from feeling overwhelmed at the amount to cover.

STEP 3: GATHER YOUR TOOLS

Decide what study method works best for you. Do you prefer to highlight in the book as you study and then go back over the highlighted portions? Or do you type out notes of the important information? Or is it helpful to make flashcards that you can carry with you? Assemble the pens, index cards, highlighters, post-it notes, and any other materials you may need so you won't be distracted by getting up to find things while you study.

If you're having a hard time retaining the information or organizing your notes, experiment with different methods. For example, try color-coding by subject with colored pens, highlighters, or post-it notes. If you learn better by hearing, try recording yourself reading your notes so you can listen while in the car, working out, or simply sitting at your desk. Ask a friend to quiz you from your flashcards, or try teaching someone the material to solidify it in your mind.

STEP 4: CREATE YOUR ENVIRONMENT

It's important to avoid distractions while you study. This includes both the obvious distractions like visitors and the subtle distractions like an uncomfortable chair (or a too-comfortable couch that makes you want to fall asleep). Set up the best study environment possible: good lighting and a comfortable work area. If background music helps you focus, you may want to turn it on, but otherwise keep the room quiet. If you are using a computer to take notes, be sure you don't have any other windows open, especially applications like social media, games, or anything else that could distract you. Silence your phone and turn off notifications. Be sure to keep water close by so you stay hydrated while you study (but avoid unhealthy drinks and snacks).

Also, take into account the best time of day to study. Are you freshest first thing in the morning? Try to set aside some time then to work through the material. Is your mind clearer in the afternoon or evening? Schedule your study session then. Another method is to study at the same time of day that you will take the test, so that your brain gets used to working on the material at that time and will be ready to focus at test time.

STEP 5: STUDY!

Once you have done all the study preparation, it's time to settle into the actual studying. Sit down, take a few moments to settle your mind so you can focus, and begin to follow your study plan. Don't give in to distractions or let yourself procrastinate. This is your time to prepare so you'll be ready to fearlessly approach the test. Make the most of the time and stay focused.

Of course, you don't want to burn out. If you study too long you may find that you're not retaining the information very well. Take regular study breaks. For example, taking five minutes out of every hour to walk briskly, breathing deeply and swinging your arms, can help your mind stay fresh.

As you get to the end of each chapter or section, it's a good idea to do a quick review. Remind yourself of what you learned and work on any difficult parts. When you feel that you've mastered the material, move on to the next part. At the end of your study session, briefly skim through your notes again.

But while review is helpful, cramming last minute is NOT. If at all possible, work ahead so that you won't need to fit all your study into the last day. Cramming overloads your brain with more information than it can process and retain, and your tired mind may struggle to recall even previously learned information when it is overwhelmed with last-minute study. Also, the urgent nature of cramming and the stress placed on your brain contribute to anxiety. You'll be more likely to go to the test feeling unprepared and having trouble thinking clearly.

So don't cram, and don't stay up late before the test, even just to review your notes at a leisurely pace. Your brain needs rest more than it needs to go over the information again. In fact, plan to finish your studies by noon or early afternoon the day before the test. Give your brain the rest of the day to relax or focus on other things, and get a good night's sleep. Then you will be fresh for the test and better able to recall what you've studied.

STEP 6: TAKE A PRACTICE TEST

Many courses offer sample tests, either online or in the study materials. This is an excellent resource to check whether you have mastered the material, as well as to prepare for the test format and environment.

Check the test format ahead of time: the number of questions, the type (multiple choice, free response, etc.), and the time limit. Then create a plan for working through them. For example, if you have 30 minutes to take a 60-question test, your limit is 30 seconds per question. Spend less time on the questions you know well so that you can take more time on the difficult ones.

If you have time to take several practice tests, take the first one open book, with no time limit. Work through the questions at your own pace and make sure you fully understand them. Gradually work up to taking a test under test conditions: sit at a desk with all study materials put away and set a timer. Pace yourself to make sure you finish the test with time to spare and go back to check your answers if you have time.

After each test, check your answers. On the questions you missed, be sure you understand why you missed them. Did you misread the question (tests can use tricky wording)? Did you forget the information? Or was it something you hadn't learned? Go back and study any shaky areas that the practice tests reveal.

Taking these tests not only helps with your grade, but also aids in combating test anxiety. If you're already used to the test conditions, you're less likely to worry about it, and working through tests until you're scoring well gives you a confidence boost. Go through the practice tests until you feel comfortable, and then you can go into the test knowing that you're ready for it.

Test Tips

On test day, you should be confident, knowing that you've prepared well and are ready to answer the questions. But aside from preparation, there are several test day strategies you can employ to maximize your performance.

First, as stated before, get a good night's sleep the night before the test (and for several nights before that, if possible). Go into the test with a fresh, alert mind rather than staying up late to study.

Try not to change too much about your normal routine on the day of the test. It's important to eat a nutritious breakfast, but if you normally don't eat breakfast at all, consider eating just a protein bar. If you're a coffee drinker, go ahead and have your normal coffee. Just make sure you time it so that the caffeine doesn't wear off right in the middle of your test. Avoid sugary beverages, and drink enough water to stay hydrated but not so much that you need a restroom break 10 minutes into the test. If your test isn't first thing in the morning, consider going for a walk or doing a light workout before the test to get your blood flowing.

Allow yourself enough time to get ready, and leave for the test with plenty of time to spare so you won't have the anxiety of scrambling to arrive in time. Another reason to be early is to select a good seat. It's helpful to sit away from doors and windows, which can be distracting. Find a good seat, get out your supplies, and settle your mind before the test begins.

When the test begins, start by going over the instructions carefully, even if you already know what to expect. Make sure you avoid any careless mistakes by following the directions.

Then begin working through the questions, pacing yourself as you've practiced. If you're not sure on an answer, don't spend too much time on it, and don't let it shake your confidence. Either skip it and come back later, or eliminate as many wrong answers as possible and guess among the remaining ones. Don't dwell on these questions as you continue—put them out of your mind and focus on what lies ahead.

Be sure to read all of the answer choices, even if you're sure the first one is the right answer. Sometimes you'll find a better one if you keep reading. But don't second-guess yourself if you do immediately know the answer. Your gut instinct is usually right. Don't let test anxiety rob you of the information you know.

If you have time at the end of the test (and if the test format allows), go back and review your answers. Be cautious about changing any, since your first instinct tends to be correct, but make sure you didn't misread any of the questions or accidentally mark the wrong answer choice. Look over any you skipped and make an educated guess.

At the end, leave the test feeling confident. You've done your best, so don't waste time worrying about your performance or wishing you could change anything. Instead, celebrate the successful completion of this test. And finally, use this test to learn how to deal with anxiety even better next time.

> **Review Video: Test Anxiety**
> Visit mometrix.com/academy and enter code: 100340

Important Qualification

Not all anxiety is created equal. If your test anxiety is causing major issues in your life beyond the classroom or testing center, or if you are experiencing troubling physical symptoms related to your anxiety, it may be a sign of a serious physiological or psychological condition. If this sounds like your situation, we strongly encourage you to seek professional help.

Additional Bonus Material

Due to our efforts to try to keep this book to a manageable length, we've created a link that will give you access to all of your additional bonus material:

mometrix.com/bonus948/emt